# Drug Facts

made

## Incredibly Quick!™

**Waterproof**
*Write on the pages
Remove old in*
*alcohol wip*

## LIPPINCOTT WILLIAMS & WILKINS
### A **Wolters Kluwer** Company

Philadelphia · Baltimore · New York · London
Buenos Aires · Hong Kong · Sydney · Tokyo

## Staff

**Executive Publisher**
Judith A. Schilling McCann, RN, MSN

**Editorial Director**
David Moreau

**Clinical Director**
Joan M. Robinson, RN, MSN

**Clinical Manager**
Eileen Cassin Gallen, RN, BSN

**Senior Art Director**
Arlene Putterman

**Art Director**
Mary Ludwicki

**Editorial Project Manager**
Jaime Stockslager Buss

**Clinical Project Manager**
Collette Bishop Hendler, RN, BS, CCRN

**Clinical Editor**
Joanne M. Bartelmo, RN, MSN

**Editors**
Karen C. Comerford, Doris Weinstock

**Copy Editor**
Kimberly Bilotta (supervisor), Amy Furman,
Pamela Wingrod

**Designer**
Lynn Foulk

**Illustrator**
Bot Roda

**Digital Composition Services**
Diane Paluba (manager), Joyce Rossi Biletz

**Manufacturing**
Patricia K. Dorshaw (director), Beth J. Welsh

**Editorial Assistants**
Megan L. Aldinger, Karen J. Kirk,
Linda K. Ruhf

**Indexer**
Karen C. Comerford

Printed in China.

DFIQ010805 — D N O S A
07 06 05    10 9 8 7 6 5 4 3 2 1

ISBN: 1-58255-796-9

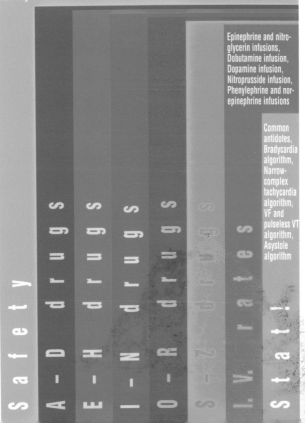

Common abbreviations, Dangerous abbreviations, Safe drug administration guidelines, Pregnancy risk categories, Therapeutic drug monitoring, Dosage calculation formulas and common conversions, Herb-drug interactions

Epinephrine and nitroglycerin infusions, Dobutamine infusion, Dopamine infusion, Nitroprusside infusion, Phenylephrine and norepinephrine infusions

Common antidotes, Bradycardia algorithm, Narrow-complex tachycardia algorithm, VF and pulseless VT algorithm, Asystole algorithm

Safety

A–D drugs

E–H drugs

I–N drugs

O–R drugs

S–Z drugs

I.V. rates

Stat!

# Common abbreviations

| | | | | |
|---|---|---|---|---|
| ACE | angiotensin-converting enzyme | | lb | pound |
| ADH | antidiuretic hormone | | LD | lactate dehydrogenase |
| AIDS | acquired immunodeficiency syndrome | | LDL | low-density lipoprotein |
| ALT | alanine transaminase | | M | molar |
| AST | aspartate transaminase | | $m^2$ | square meter |
| b.i.d. | twice daily | | MAO | monoamine oxidase |
| BSA | body surface area | | mcg | microgram |
| BUN | blood urea nitrogen | | mEq | milliequivalent |
| CBC | complete blood count | | mg | milligram |
| CK | creatine kinase | | MI | myocardial infarction |
| CMV | cytomegalovirus | | min | minute |
| CNS | central nervous system | | ml | milliliter |
| COPD | chronic obstructive pulmonary disease | | $mm^3$ | cubic millimeter |
| CSF | cerebrospinal fluid | | msec | millisecond |
| CV | cardiovascular | | NSAID | nonsteroidal anti-inflammatory drug |
| $D_5W$ | dextrose 5% in water | | OTC | over-the-counter |
| DIC | disseminated intravascular coagulation | | PCA | patient-controlled analgesia |
| dl | deciliter | | P.O. | by mouth |
| ECG | electrocardiogram | | P.R. | by rectum |
| EEG | electroencephalogram | | p.r.n. | as needed |
| g | gram | | PT | prothrombin time |
| G | gauge | | PTT | partial thromboplastin time |
| GFR | glomerular filtration rate | | PVC | premature ventricular contraction |
| GI | gastrointestinal | | q | every |
| gtt | drops | | q.i.d. | four times daily |
| GU | genitourinary | | RBC | red blood cell |
| $h_1$ | histamine-1 | | RSV | respiratory syncytial virus |
| $h_2$ | histamine-2 | | sec | second |
| HDL | high-density lipoprotein | | SIADH | syndrome of inappropriate antidiuretic hormone |
| HIV | human immunodeficiency virus | | S.L. | sublingual |
| I.D. | intradermal | | SSRI | selective serotonin reuptake inhibitor |
| I.M. | intramuscular | | SubQ | subcutaneous |
| INR | International Normalized Ratio | | $T_3$ | triiodothyronine |
| IPPB | intermittent positive-pressure breathing | | $T_4$ | thyroxine |
| I.V. | intravenous | | TCA | tricyclic antidepressant |
| kg | kilogram | | t.i.d. | three times daily |
| L | liter | | tsp | teaspoon |
| | | | USP | United States Pharmacopeia |
| | | | UTI | urinary tract infection |
| | | | WBC | white blood cell |

## Dangerous abbreviations

The Joint Commission on Accreditation of Healthcare Organizations has approved the following "minimum required list" of dangerous abbreviations, acronyms, and symbols that shouldn't be used by accredited organizations. They have also provided a list of other abbreviations that medical personnel should consider not using. Avoiding use of all of these abbreviations, acronyms, and symbols should help protect patients from the effects of miscommunication in clinical documentation.

### Minimum required list

| Abbreviation | Potential problem | Preferred term |
|---|---|---|
| U (for unit) | Mistaken as zero, four, or cc | Write "unit." |
| IU (for international unit) | Mistaken as IV (intravenous) or 10 | Write "international unit." |
| Q.D., Q.O.D. (Latin abbreviations for "once daily" and "every other day") | Mistaken for each other; the period after the "Q" can be mistaken for an "I"; the "O" can also be mistaken for an "I" | Write "daily" and "every other day." |
| Trailing zero (X.0 mg); lack of leading zero (.X mg) | Decimal point is missed | Never write a zero by itself after a decimal point (X mg); always use a zero before a decimal point (0.X mg). |
| MS, $MSO_4$, $MgSO_4$ | Confused with each other | Write "morphine sulfate" or "magnesium sulfate." |

Other dangerous abbreviations

| Abbreviation | Potential problem | Preferred term |
|---|---|---|
| µg (for microgram) | Mistaken for mg (milligram), resulting in overdose | Write "mcg." |
| H.S. (for half-strength or Latin abbreviation for "bedtime") | Mistaken for either "half-strength" or "hour of sleep"; "q H.S." mistaken for "every hour" | Write "half-strength" or "at bedtime." |
| T.I.W. (for three times a week) | Mistaken for "three times a day" or "twice weekly" | Write "3 times weekly" or "three times weekly." |
| S.C. or S.Q. (for subcutaneous) | Mistaken for "SL" (sublingual) or "5 every" | Write "sub-Q," "subQ," or "subcutaneously." |
| D/C (for discharge) | Mistaken for discontinue whatever drugs follow | Write "discharge." |
| c.c. (for cubic centimeter) | Mistaken for U (units) when written poorly | Write "ml" (milliliter). |
| A.S., A.D., A.U. (Latin abbreviations for "left ear," "right ear," and "both ears") | Mistaken for OS, OD, OU | Write "left ear," "right ear," or "both ears." |

## Safe drug administration guidelines

When administering a drug, be sure to adhere to best practices to avoid potential problems. You can help prevent drug mistakes by following these guidelines as well as your facility's policies.

### Drug orders

• Don't rely on the pharmacy computer system to detect all unsafe orders. Before you give a drug, understand the correct dosage, indications, and adverse effects. If necessary, check a current drug reference guide.

• Be aware of the drugs your patient takes regularly, and question any deviation from his regular routine. As with any drug, take your time and read the label carefully.

• Ask all prescribers to spell out drug names and any error-prone abbreviations.

• Before you give drugs that are ordered in units, such as insulin and heparin, always check the prescriber's written order against the provided dose. Never abbreviate the word "units."

• If you must accept a verbal order, have another nurse listen in; then transcribe that order directly onto an order form and repeat it to the prescriber to ensure that you've transcribed it correctly.

• To prevent an acetaminophen overdose from combined analgesics, note the amount of acetaminophen in each drug. Beware of substitutions by the pharmacy because the amount of acetaminophen may vary.

• Keep in mind that lipid-based products have different dosages than their conventional counterparts. Check the doctor's orders and labels carefully to avoid confusion.

### Drug preparation

• If a familiar drug has an unfamiliar appearance, find out why. If the pharmacist cites a manufacturing change, ask him to double-check whether he has received verification from the manufacturer. Document the appearance discrepancy, your actions, and the pharmacist's response in the patient record.

• Obtain a new allergy history with each admission. If the patient's history must be faxed, name the drugs, note how many are included, and follow your facility's faxing safeguards. If the pharmacy also adheres to strict guidelines, the computer-generated medication administration record should be accurate.

### Giving drugs

• Use two patient identifiers, such as the patient's name and assigned medical record number, to identify the patient before administering any drug or treatment. Teach the patient to offer his identification bracelet for inspection when anyone arrives with drugs and to insist on having it replaced if it's removed.

• Ask the patient about his use of alternative therapies, including herbs, and record your findings in his medical record. Monitor the patient carefully and report unusual events. Ask the patient to keep a diary of all therapies he uses and to take the diary for review each time he visits a health care professional.

### Calculation errors

• Writing the mg/kg or mg/m$^2$ dose and the calculated dose provides a safeguard against calculation errors. Whenever a prescriber provides the calculation, double-check it and document that the dose was verified.
• Don't assume that liquid drugs are less likely to cause harm than other forms, including parenteral ones. Pediatric and geriatric patients commonly receive liquid drugs and may be especially sensitive to the effects of an inaccurate dose. If a unit-dose form isn't available, calculate carefully and double-check your math and the drug label.
• Leaving potentially dangerous chemicals near a patient is extremely risky, especially when the container labels don't indicate toxicity. To prevent problems, never leave drug containers near a patient.
• Read the label on every drug you prepare and never administer any drug that isn't labeled.

### Dosage equations

• After you calculate a drug dosage, always have another nurse calculate it independently to double-check your results. If doubts or questions remain or if the calculations don't match, ask a pharmacist to calculate the dose before you give the drug.

### Air bubbles in pump tubing

• To clear bubbles from I.V. tubing, never increase the pump's flow rate to flush the line. Instead, remove the tubing from the pump, disconnect it from the patient, and use the flow-control clamp to establish gravity flow.
• When the bubbles have been removed, return the tubing to the pump, restart the infusion, and recheck the flow rate.

### Incorrect administration route

• When a patient has multiple I.V. lines, label the distal end of each line.
• Using a parenteral syringe to prepare oral liquid drugs increases the chance for error because the syringe tip fits easily into I.V. ports. To safely give an oral drug through a feeding tube, use a dose prepared by the pharmacy and a syringe with the appropriate tip.

## Pregnancy risk categories

Pregnancy risk categories were designed to alert prescribers to the risks associated with drugs administered during pregnancy. The categories include:

• **A:** Adequate studies in pregnant women have failed to show a risk to the fetus.

• **B:** Animal studies haven't shown a risk to the fetus, but controlled studies haven't been conducted in pregnant women; or animal studies have shown an adverse effect on the fetus, but adequate studies in pregnant women haven't shown a risk to the fetus.

• **C:** Animal studies have shown an adverse effect on the fetus, but adequate studies haven't been conducted in humans. The benefits from use in pregnant women may be acceptable despite potential risks.

• **D:** The drug may cause risk to the fetus, but the potential benefits of use in pregnant women may be acceptable despite the risks (such as in life-threatening situations or serious diseases for which safer drugs can't be used or are ineffective).

• **X:** Studies in animals and humans show fetal abnormalities, or adverse reaction reports indicate evidence of fetal risk. The risks involved clearly outweigh potential benefits.

• **NR:** Not rated.

# Therapeutic drug monitoring

| Drug | Laboratory test | Therapeutic range |
|------|-----------------|-------------------|
| amikacin | amikacin peak | 20-30 mcg/ml (SI, 34-52 μmol/L) |
| | amikacin trough | 1-8 mcg/ml (SI, 2-14 μmol/L) |
| amiodarone | amiodarone level | 0.5-2.5 mg/L (SI, 0.8-3.9 μmol/L) |
| digoxin | digoxin level | 0.8-2 ng/ml (SI, 1-2.6 mol/L) |
| gentamicin | gentamicin peak | 4-10 mcg/ml (SI, 8-21 μmol/L) |
| | gentamicin trough | 0.5-2 mcg/ml (SI, 1-4 μmol/L) |
| lithium | lithium level | 0.6-1.2 mEq/L (SI, 0.6-1.2 mmol/L) |
| phenytoin | phenytoin level | 10-20 mcg/ml (SI, 40-70 μmol/L) |
| procainamide | procainamide | 4-10 mcg/ml (SI, 17-42 μmol/L) |
| | N-acetylprocainamide (NAPA) | 10-30 mcg/ml (SI, 42-127 μmol/L) |
| theophylline | theophylline level | 10-20 mcg/ml (SI, 56-111 μmol/L) |
| vancomycin | vancomycin peak | 25-40 mcg/ml (SI, 17-27 μmol/L) |
| | vancomycin trough | 5-10 mcg/ml (SI, 3.4-6.8 μmol/L) |

## Dosage calculation formulas and common conversions

### Common calculations

$$\text{Body surface area in m}^2 = \sqrt{\frac{\text{height in cm} \times \text{weight in kg}}{3{,}600}}$$

$$\text{mcg/ml} = \text{mg/ml} \times 1{,}000$$

$$\text{ml/minute} = \frac{\text{ml/hour}}{60}$$

$$\text{gtt/minute} = \frac{\text{volume in ml to be infused}}{\text{time in minutes}} \times \text{drip factor in gtt/ml}$$

$$\text{mg/minute} = \frac{\text{mg in bag}}{\text{ml in bag}} \times \text{flow rate} \div 60$$

$$\text{mcg/minute} = \frac{\text{mg in bag}}{\text{ml in bag}} \div 0.06 \times \text{flow rate}$$

$$\text{mcg/kg/minute} = \frac{\text{mcg/ml} \times \text{ml/minute}}{\text{weight in kg}}$$

### Common conversions

| | | |
|---|---|---|
| 1 kg = 1,000 g | 1 L = 1,000 ml | 8 oz = 240 ml |
| 1 g = 1,000 mg | 1 ml = 1,000 microliters (µl) | 1 oz = 28 g |
| 1 mg = 1,000 mcg | 1 tsp = 5 ml | 1 lb = 454 g |
| | 1 tbs = 15 ml | 2.2 lb = 1 kg |
| 1″ = 2.54 cm | 2 tbs = 30 ml | |

# Herb-drug Interactions

| Herb | Drug | Possible effects |
|---|---|---|
| echinacea | hepatotoxic drugs | May increase risk of liver damage |
| | immunosuppressants | Herb may counteract drugs |
| ginkgo | warfarin | Increases bleeding time without increased INR |
| | anticoagulants, antiplatelets | May lead to increased anticoagulation |
| | anticonvulsants | May decrease effectiveness of drugs |
| | drugs known to lower seizure threshold | May further reduce seizure threshold |
| | insulin | Ginkgo leaf extract can affect glucose level |
| | thiazide diuretics | Ginkgo leaf may increase blood pressure |
| ginseng | anabolic steroids, hormones | May potentiate effects of drugs |
| | antibiotics | May enhance effects of some antibiotics |
| | anticoagulants, antiplatelets | Decrease platelet adhesiveness |
| | antidiabetics | May enhance glucose-lowering effects |
| | digoxin | May falsely elevate drug level |
| | furosemide | May decrease diuretic effect |
| | warfarin | May reverse drug effects |
| kava | benzodiazepines | Concurrent use may result in comalike state |
| | hepatotoxic drugs | May increase the risk of liver damage |
| | levodopa | Decreases effectiveness of drug |

# Herb-drug interactions (continued)

| Herb | Drug | Possible effects |
|------|------|------------------|
| St. John's wort | cyclosporine | Reduces drug levels below therapeutic levels |
| | digoxin | Decreases therapeutic effects of drug |
| | HIV protease inhibitors, indinavir, nonnucleoside reverse transcriptase inhibitors | Decrease therapeutic effects of drug |
| | hormonal contraceptives | Decrease effects of drug |
| | theophylline | Decreases effects of drug |
| | warfarin | Decreases effects of drug |

# abciximab (ab-SIKS-ih-mahb)

ReoPro

Pregnancy risk category: C

## Indications and dosages

**Adjunct to percutaneous translu-minal coronary angioplasty (PTCA) or atherectomy to prevent acute cardiac ischemic complications in patients at high risk for abrupt closure of treated coronary vessel**

■ *Adults:* 0.25 mg/kg as an I.V. bolus given 10 to 60 minutes before start of PTCA or atherecto-my; then a continuous I.V. infusion of 0.125 mcg/kg/minute to a maxi-mum of 10 mcg/minute for 12 hours.

**Unstable angina not responding to conventional medical therapy in patients scheduled for percuta-neous coronary intervention within 24 hours**

■ *Adults:* 0.25 mg/kg as an I.V. bolus; then an 18- to 24-hour infu-sion of 10 mcg/minute concluding 1 hour after percutaneous coronary intervention.

## Adverse reactions

Abdominal pain • abnormal vision • anemia • **bleeding** • **bradycardia** • confusion • headache • hyper-esthesia • hypoesthesia • *hypo-tension* • leukocytosis • *nausea* • pain • peripheral edema • pleural effusion • pleurisy • pneumonia • **thrombocytopenia** • vomiting

## Nursing considerations

■ Inspect solution for particulate matter before I.V. administration. If opaque particles are visible, discard solution and obtain new vial.

■ Withdraw needed amount of drug for I.V. bolus through a sterile, nonpyogenic, low-protein-binding 0.2- or 0.22-micron filter into a syringe. Give I.V. bolus 10 to 60 minutes before procedure.

■ Withdraw needed amount of drug for continuous I.V. infusion through a sterile, nonpyogenic, low-protein-binding 0.2- or 0.22-micron filter into a syringe. Inject into 250 ml of sterile normal saline solution or $D_5W$, and infuse at 0.125 mcg/kg/minute to a maxi-mum of 10 mcg/minute for 12 hours via a continuous infusion pump equipped with an in-line filter. Discard unused portion at end of 12-hour infusion.

■ Give drug in a separate I.V. line whenever possible; add no other drug to the infusion solution.

*Alert:* Keep epinephrine, dopamine, theophylline, antihistamines, and corticosteroids readily available in case of anaphylaxis.

■ Monitor patient closely for bleed-ing at the arterial access site and internal bleeding involving the GI or GU tract or retroperitoneal sites.

## abciximab (continued)

■ Institute bleeding precautions. Keep patient on bed rest for 6 to 8 hours after sheath removal or end of drug infusion, whichever is later. Minimize or avoid, if possible, arterial and venous punctures, I.M. injections, urinary catheters, nasogastric tubes, automatic blood pressure cuffs, and nasotracheal intubation.

■ During abciximab infusion, remove sheath only after heparin has been stopped and its effects largely reversed.

■ Obtain platelet count before treatment, 2 to 4 hours after bolus dose, and 24 hours after bolus dose or before discharge, whichever is first.

■ Anticipate stopping abciximab and giving platelets for severe bleeding or thrombocytopenia.

**Watch out!** Don't confuse abciximab with arcitumomab.

# acetaminophen (ah-see-tuh-MIH-nuh-fin)

Abenol*, Acephen, Aceta, Acetaminophen, Actamin, Aminofen, Apacet, Apo-Acetaminophen*, Atasol*, Banesin, Dapa, Exdol*, FeverAll, Genapap, Genebs, Liquiprin, Neopap, Oraphen-PD, Panadol, Redutemp, Robigesic*, Rounox*, Snaplets-FR, St. Joseph Aspirin-free Fever Reducer for Children, Suppap, Tapanol, Tempra, Tylenol, Valorin

Pregnancy risk category: B

## Indications and dosages

### Mild pain or fever

**PO.**

■ **Adults:** 325 to 650 mg PO, q 4 to 6 hours; or 1 g PO, t.i.d. or q.i.d., p.r.n. Or, two extended-release caplets PO, q 8 hours. Maximum, 4 g daily. For long-term therapy, don't exceed 2.6 g daily unless prescribed and monitored closely by health care provider.

■ **Children older than age 14:** 650 mg PO, q 4 to 6 hours, p.r.n.

■ **Children ages 12 to 14:** 640 mg PO, q 4 to 6 hours, p.r.n.

■ **Children age 11:** 480 mg PO, q 4 to 6 hours, p.r.n.

■ **Children ages 9 to 10:** 400 mg PO, q 4 to 6 hours, p.r.n.

■ **Children ages 6 to 8:** 320 mg PO, q 4 to 6 hours, p.r.n.

■ **Children ages 4 to 5:** 240 mg PO, q 4 to 6 hours, p.r.n.

■ **Children ages 2 to 3:** 160 mg PO, q 4 to 6 hours, p.r.n.

■ **Children ages 12 to 24 months:** 120 mg PO, q 4 to 6 hours, p.r.n.

■ **Children ages 4 to 12 months:** 80 mg PO, q 4 to 6 hours, p.r.n.

■ **Children up to age 4 months:** 40 mg PO, q 4 to 6 hours, p.r.n. Or, 10 to 15 mg/kg/dose q 4 hours.

**PR.**

■ **Adults:** 650 mg PR, q 4 to 6 hours, p.r.n. Don't exceed five doses in 24 hours.

■ **Children ages 6 to 12:** 325 mg PR, q 4 to 6 hours, p.r.n.

■ **Children ages 3 to 6:** 120 to 125 mg PR, q 4 to 6 hours, p.r.n.

■ **Children ages 1 to 3:** 80 mg PR, q 4 to 6 hours, p.r.n.

■ **Children ages 3 to 12 months:** 80 mg PR, q 6 hours, p.r.n.

## Adverse reactions

Hemolytic anemia • **hypoglycemia** • jaundice • **leukopenia** • liver **damage** • **neutropenia** • **pancyto-penia** • rash • urticaria

## Nursing considerations

■ Use cautiously in patients with histories of long-term alcohol use because therapeutic dosages cause hepatotoxicity.

*Alert:* Be aware that many OTC and prescription products contain acetaminophen.

12

# acetylcysteine (ah-see-til-SIS-teen)

Acetadote, Mucomyst, Mucosil-10, Mucosil-20

Pregnancy risk category: **B**

## Indications and dosages

**Adjunct therapy for abnormal viscid or inspissated mucus secretions in patients with pneumonia, bronchitis, bronchiectasis, primary amyloidosis of the lung, tuberculosis, cystic fibrosis, emphysema, atelectasis, pulmonary complications of thoracic surgery, or CV surgery**
■ *Adults and children:* 1 to 2 ml 10% or 20% solution by direct instillation into trachea as often as q hour. Or, 1 to 10 ml of 20% solution or 2 to 20 ml of 10% solution by nebulization q 2 to 6 hours, p.r.n.

**Acetaminophen toxicity**
■ *Adults and children:* Initially, 140 mg/kg P.O.; then 70 mg/kg P.O. q 4 hours for 17 doses (total). Or, a loading dose of 150 mg/kg I.V. over 15 minutes; then I.V. maintenance dose of 50 mg/kg infused over 4 hours, followed by 100 mg/kg infused over 16 hours.

## Adverse reactions

Abnormal thinking ▪ *anaphylactoid reaction* ▪ **angioedema** ▪ **bronchospasm** ▪ chest tightness ▪ chills ▪ clamminess ▪ cough ▪ diaphoresis ▪ drowsiness ▪ dyspnea ▪ ear pain ▪ eye pain ▪ fever ▪ flushing ▪ gait disturbance ▪ hypertension ▪ hypotension ▪ *nausea* ▪ pharyngitis ▪ pruritus ▪ rash ▪ *rhinorrhea* ▪ rhonchi ▪ *stomatitis* ▪ tachycardia ▪ throat tightness ▪ urticaria ▪ *vomiting*

## Nursing considerations

■ Use plastic, glass, stainless steel, or another nonreactive metal when giving by nebulization.
■ Drug is physically or chemically incompatible with tetracyclines, erythromycin lactobionate, amphotericin B, and ampicillin sodium. If given by aerosol inhalation, nebulize these drugs separately. Iodized oil, trypsin, and hydrogen peroxide are physically incompatible with acetylcysteine; don't add to nebulizer.
■ Drug smells strongly of sulfur. Mixing oral form with juice or cola improves its palatability.
■ Drug delivered through nasogastric tube may be diluted with water.
■ Monitor cough type and frequency.
*Alert:* Monitor patient for bronchospasm, especially if he has asthma.
■ Use fresh dilutions within 1 hour. Store undiluted solutions that have been opened in the refrigerator for up to 96 hours.
■ Ingestion of more than 150 mg/kg of acetaminophen may cause hepa-

# acetylcysteine (continued)

toxicity. Measure acetaminophen level 4 hours after ingestion to determine risk of hepatotoxicity.

**Alert:** Acetylcysteine is used to treat acetaminophen overdose within 24 hours after ingestion. Start treatment immediately as prescribed; don't wait for results of acetaminophen level. Acetadote I.V. should be given within 10 hours after acetaminophen ingestion to minimize hepatic injury.

■ If you suspect acetaminophen overdose, get baseline PT and AST, ALT, bilirubin, BUN, creatinine, glucose, and electrolyte levels.

■ Dilute oral doses used in treating acetaminophen overdose with cola, fruit juice, or water before administration. Dilute the 20% solution to 5% solution (add 3 ml of diluent to each milliliter of acetylcysteine). If patient vomits within 1 hour of receiving loading or maintenance dose, repeat dose. Use diluted solution within 1 hour.

**Alert:** Monitor patient receiving I.V. acetylcysteine for anaphylactoid reactions.

■ Be aware that facial erythema may occur within 30 to 60 minutes after the start of an I.V. infusion and usually resolves without infusion interruption.

■ When acetaminophen level drops below toxic level according to nomogram, acetylcysteine therapy may be stopped.

**Watch out!** Don't confuse acetylcysteine with acetylcholine.

## activated charcoal (AK-tih-vay-ted CHAR-kohl)

Actidose, Actidose-Aqua, Actidose with Sorbitol, CharcoAid, CharcoAid 2000, CharcoCaps, Liqui-Char

Pregnancy risk category: C

### Indications and dosages

**Flatulence, dyspepsia**
■ *Adults:* 600 mg to 5 g P.O. as single dose or 0.975 to 3.9 g P.O. t.i.d. after meals.

**Poisoning**
■ *Adults and children:* Initially, 1 to 2 g/kg (30 to 100 g) P.O. or 10 times the amount of poison ingested as a suspension in 120 to 240 ml (4 to 8 oz) of water.

### Adverse reactions

*Black stools* • constipation • ***intestinal obstruction*** • nausea

### Nursing considerations

■ Although there are no known contraindications, drug isn't effective for treating all acute poisonings.
*Alert:* Drug is commonly used for treating poisoning or overdose with acetaminophen, aspirin, atropine, barbiturates, dextropropoxyphene, digoxin, poisonous mushrooms, oxalic acid, phenol, phenytoin, propantheline, propoxyphene, strychnine, or TCAs. Check with poison control center for use in other types of poisonings or overdose.
■ For maximal effect, give within 30 minutes after poison ingestion.

■ Mix powder (most effective form) with tap water to consistency of thick syrup. Adding a small amount of fruit juice or flavoring makes mix more palatable. Don't mix with ice cream, milk, or sherbet because these substances decrease the adsorptive capacity of activated charcoal.
*Alert:* Don't aspirate or allow patient to aspirate charcoal powder; aspirating the powder has resulted in death.
■ Give by large-bore nasogastric tube after lavage, if needed.
■ If patient vomits shortly after administration, be prepared to repeat dose.
■ Space doses at least 1 hour apart from other drugs if treatment is for indications other than poisoning.
■ Follow treatment with stool softener or laxative to prevent constipation unless sorbitol is part of product ingredients.
■ Don't use charcoal with sorbitol in fructose-intolerant patients or in children younger than age 1.
*Alert:* Drug is ineffective for poisoning or overdose of cyanide, mineral acids, caustic alkalis, and organic solvents. It's minimally effective for overdose of ethanol, lithium, methanol, and iron salts.
**Watch out!** Don't confuse Actidose with Actos.

## acyclovir (ay-SIGH-kloh-veer)

acyclovir
**Avirax†, Zovirax**
acyclovir sodium
**Avirax†, Zovirax**

Pregnancy risk category: C

## Indications and dosages

**First and recurrent episodes of mucocutaneous herpes simplex virus (HSV-1 and HSV-2) infections in immunocompromised patients; severe first episodes of genital herpes in patients who aren't immunocompromised**

■ *Adults and children age 12 and older:* 5 mg/kg given I.V. over 1 hour q 8 hours for 7 days. Give for 5 to 7 days for severe first episode of genital herpes.

■ *Children younger than age 12:* 10 mg/kg given I.V. over 1 hour q 8 hours for 7 days.

**First genital herpes episode**

■ *Adults:* 200 mg P.O. q 4 hours while awake, five times daily; or 400 mg P.O. q 8 hours. Continue for 7 to 10 days.

**Intermittent therapy for recurrent genital herpes**

■ *Adults:* 200 mg P.O. q 4 hours while awake, five times daily. Continue for 5 days. Begin therapy at first sign of recurrence.

**Long-term suppressive therapy for recurrent genital herpes**

■ *Adults:* 400 mg P.O. b.i.d. for up to 12 months. Or, 200 mg P.O. three to five times daily for up to 12 months.

**Varicella (chickenpox) infections in immunocompromised patients**

■ *Adults and children age 12 and older:* 10 mg/kg I.V. over 1 hour q 8 hours for 7 days. Dosage for obese patients is 10 mg/kg based on ideal body weight q 8 hours for 7 days. Don't exceed maximum dosage equivalent of 20 mg/kg q 8 hours.

■ *Children younger than age 12:* 20 mg/kg I.V. over 1 hour q 8 hours for 7 days.

**Varicella infection in immunocompetent patients**

■ *Adults and children weighing more than 40 kg (88 lb):* 800 mg P.O. q.i.d. for 5 days.

■ *Children age 2 and older weighing less than 40 kg:* 20 mg/kg (maximum 800 mg/dose) P.O. q.i.d. for 5 days. Start therapy as soon as symptoms appear.

**Acute herpes zoster infection in immunocompetent patients**

■ *Adults and children age 12 and older:* 800 mg P.O. q 4 hours five times daily for 7 to 10 days.

**Herpes simplex encephalitis**

■ *Adults and children age 12 and older:* 10 mg/kg I.V. over 1 hour q 8 hours for 10 days.

■ *Children ages 3 months to 12 years:* 20 mg/kg I.V. over 1 hour q 8 hours for 10 days.

## acyclovir *(continued)*

### Neonatal herpes simplex virus infection

■ *Neonates to age 3 months:*
10 mg/kg I.V. over 1 hour q 8 hours for 10 days.

*Adjust-a-dose:* For patients receiving the I.V. form, if creatinine clearance is 25 to 50 ml/minute, give 100% of dose q 12 hours; if clearance is 10 to 24 ml/minute, give 100% of dose q 24 hours; if clearance is less than 10 ml/minute, give 50% of dose q 24 hours.

For patients receiving the P.O. form, if normal dose is 200 mg q 4 hours five times daily and creatinine clearance is less than 10 ml/minute, give 200 mg P.O. q 12 hours. If normal dose is 400 mg q 12 hours and clearance is less than 10 ml/minute, give 200 mg q 12 hours. If normal dose is 800 mg q 4 hours five times daily and clearance is 10 to 25 ml/minute, give 800 mg q 8 hours; if clearance is less than 10 ml/minute, give 800 mg q 12 hours.

### Adverse reactions

*Acute renal failure* • diarrhea • *encephalopathic changes* • headache • hematuria • *inflammation or phlebitis at injection site* • itching • *leukopenia* • malaise • nausea • rash • *thrombocytopenia* • thrombocytosis • urticaria • *vomiting*

### Nursing considerations

■ Use cautiously in patients with neurologic problems, renal disease, or dehydration and in those receiving other nephrotoxic drugs.

■ Give I.V. infusion over at least 1 hour to prevent renal tubular damage. Don't give by bolus injection.

■ Solutions concentrated at 7 mg/ml or more may increase the risk of phlebitis.

■ Encourage fluid intake because patient must be adequately hydrated during acyclovir infusion. Monitor intake and output, especially within the first 2 hours after I.V. administration.

*Alert:* Don't give I.M. or subQ.

■ Monitor renal function if acyclovir is used in patients with renal disease or dehydration and in those taking other nephrotoxic drugs.

**Watch out!** Don't confuse acyclovir sodium (Zovirax) vials with acetazolamide sodium (Diamox) vials, which may look alike.

**Watch out!** Don't confuse Zovirax with Zyvox.

## adenosine (uh-DEN-oh-seen)

Adenocard

Pregnancy risk category: **C**

### Indications and dosages

**To convert paroxysmal supraventricular tachycardia (PSVT) to sinus rhythm**

■ *Adults and children weighing 50 kg (110 lb) or more:* 6 mg I.V. by rapid bolus injection over 1 to 2 seconds. If PSVT isn't eliminated in 1 to 2 minutes, give 12 mg by rapid I.V. push and repeat if needed.

■ *Children weighing less than 50 kg:* Initially, 0.05 to 0.1 mg/kg I.V. by rapid bolus injection, followed by a saline flush. If PSVT isn't eliminated in 1 to 2 minutes, give additional bolus injections, increasing the amount given by 0.05- to 0.1-mg/kg increments, followed by a saline flush. Continue, p.r.n., until conversion or a maximum single dose of 0.3 mg/kg is given.

### Adverse reactions

Chest pressure ▪ dizziness ▪ *dyspnea* ▪ *facial flushing* ▪ headache ▪ light-headedness ▪ nausea ▪ numbness ▪ *shortness of breath* ▪ tingling in arms

### Nursing considerations

■ Drug is contraindicated in patients with second- or third-degree heart block or sinus node disease, except those with pacemakers.

■ Use cautiously in patients with asthma, emphysema, or bronchitis because bronchospasm may occur.

■ Give directly into a vein, if possible; when giving through an I.V. line, use port closest to the patient.

■ Flush immediately and rapidly with normal saline solution to ensure that the drug quickly reaches systemic circulation.

■ Don't give single doses exceeding 12 mg.

■ In adults, avoid giving drug through a central line because doing so may prolong asystole.

*Alert:* Because new arrhythmias, including heart block and prolonged asystole, may develop, monitor cardiac rhythm and be prepared to give appropriate therapy.

# albuterol sulfate (al-BYOO-ter-ohl SUL-fayt)

AccuNeb, Proventil, Proventil HFA, Proventil Repetabs, Ventolin, Ventolin HFA, Volmax, VoSpire ER

Pregnancy risk category: C

## Indications and dosages

**To prevent or treat bronchospasm in patients with reversible obstructive airway disease**

*Capsules for inhalation*

■ *Adults and children age 4 and older:* 200 mcg inhaled q 4 to 6 hours using a Rotahaler inhalation device. Some patients may need 400 mcg q 4 to 6 hours.

*Extended-release tablets*

■ *Adults and children older than age 12:* 4 to 8 mg P.O. q 12 hours. Maximum, 16 mg b.i.d.
■ *Children ages 6 to 12:* 4 mg P.O. q 2 hours. Maximum, 12 mg b.i.d.

*Oral tablets*

■ *Adults and children older than age 12:* 2 to 4 mg P.O. t.i.d. or q.i.d. Maximum, 8 mg q.i.d.
■ *Children ages 6 to 12:* 2 mg P.O. t.i.d. or q.i.d. Maximum, 6 mg q.i.d.

*Solution for inhalation*

■ *Adults and children older than age 12:* 2.5 mg t.i.d. or q.i.d. by nebulizer. To prepare solution, use 0.5 ml of 0.5% solution diluted with 2.5 ml of normal saline solution. Or, use 3 ml of 0.083% solution.
■ *Children ages 2 to 12:* Initially, 0.1 to 0.15 mg/kg by nebulizer, with subsequent dosage titrated to response. Don't exceed 2.5 mg t.i.d. or q.i.d. by nebulization.

*Syrup*

■ *Adults and children older than age 12:* 2 to 4 mg (1 to 2 tsp) P.O. t.i.d. or q.i.d. Maximum, 8 mg q.i.d.
■ *Children ages 6 to 12:* 2 mg (1 tsp) P.O. t.i.d. or q.i.d. Maximum, 24 mg daily in divided doses.
■ *Children ages 2 to 6:* Initially, 0.1 mg/kg P.O. t.i.d. Starting dose shouldn't exceed 2 mg (1 tsp) t.i.d. Maximum, 4 mg (2 tsp) t.i.d.
*Adjust-a-dose:* For elderly patients and those sensitive to beta stimulators, 2 mg P.O. t.i.d. or q.i.d. as oral tablets or syrup. Maximum, 8 mg t.i.d. or q.i.d.

**To prevent exercise-induced bronchospasm**

■ *Adults and children age 4 and older:* 200-mcg capsule for inhalation using a Rotahaler inhalation device 15 minutes before exercise. Or, 2 inhalations using the metered-dose inhaler 15 minutes before exercise.

## Adverse reactions

Anorexia ▪ bad taste ▪ bronchitis ▪ **bronchospasm** ▪ CNS stimulation ▪ cough ▪ dizziness ▪ dry and irritated nose and throat (inhaled form) ▪ dyspnea ▪ epistaxis ▪ *headache* ▪ heartburn ▪ hoarseness ▪ *hyperactivity* ▪ hypersensitivity reactions ▪ hypertension ▪ hypo-

*(continued)*

kalemia • increased appetite • increased sputum • insomnia • malaise • muscle cramps • nasal congestion • *nausea* • *nervousness* • *palpitations* • *tachycardia* • *tremor* • *vomiting* • weakness • wheezing

### Nursing considerations

■ Use cautiously in patients with CV disorders, hyperthyroidism, or diabetes mellitus and in those who are unusually responsive to adrenergics.

*Alert:* Patients may use tablets and aerosols together. Monitor these patients closely for signs and symptoms of toxicity.

**Watch out!** Don't confuse albuterol with atenolol or Albutein. Don't confuse Flomax with Volmax.

# alendronate sodium
(ah-LEN-droh-nayt SOH-dee-um)

Fosamax

Pregnancy risk category: C

## Indications and dosages

**Osteoporosis in postmenopausal women; to increase bone mass in men with osteoporosis**
■ *Adults:* 10 mg P.O. daily or 70-mg tablet P.O. once weekly.
**Paget's disease of bone**
■ *Adults:* 40 mg P.O. daily for 6 months.
**To prevent osteoporosis in postmenopausal women**
■ *Adults:* 5 mg P.O. daily or 35-mg tablet P.O. once weekly.
**Glucocorticoid-induced osteoporosis in men and women receiving glucocorticoids in a daily dose equivalent to 7.5 mg or more of prednisone and who have low bone mineral density**
■ *Adults:* 5 mg P.O. daily. For postmenopausal women not receiving estrogen, recommended dose is 10 mg P.O. daily.

## Adverse reactions

Abdominal distention ■ abdominal pain ■ acid regurgitation ■ constipation ■ diarrhea ■ dyspepsia ■ dysphagia ■ esophageal ulcer ■ flatulence ■ gastritis ■ headache ■ musculoskeletal pain ■ nausea ■ taste perversion ■ vomiting

## Nursing considerations

■ Drug is contraindicated in patients with hypocalcemia, severe renal insufficiency, or abnormalities of the esophagus.
■ Use cautiously in patients with dysphagia, symptomatic esophageal diseases, gastritis, duodenitis, ulcers, or mild to moderate renal insufficiency.
■ Correct hypocalcemia and other disturbances of mineral metabolism (such as vitamin D deficiency) before therapy begins.
*Alert:* Give drug with 6 to 8 oz of water at least 30 minutes before patient's first food or drink of the day, to facilitate delivery to the stomach. Don't allow patient to lie down for 30 minutes after taking drug.
■ Monitor patient's calcium and phosphate levels throughout therapy.
**Watch out!** Don't confuse Fosamax with Flomax.

# alprazolam (al-PRAH-zoh-lam)

Pregnancy risk category: D

## Indications and dosages

### Anxiety

■ **Adults:** Usual first dose, 0.25 to 0.5 mg PO, t.i.d. Maximum, 4 mg daily in divided doses.

**Elderly patients:** Usual first dose, 0.25 mg PO, b.i.d. or t.i.d. Maximum, 4 mg daily in divided doses.

### Panic disorders

■ **Adults:** 0.5 mg PO, t.i.d., increased at intervals of 3 to 4 days in increments of no more than 1 mg. Maximum, 10 mg daily in divided doses. If using extended-release tablets, start with 0.5 to 1 mg PO, once daily. Increase by no more than 1 mg q 3 to 4 days. Maximum daily dose, 10 mg.

**Adjust-a-dose:** For debilitated patients or those with advanced hepatic disease, usual first dose is 0.25 mg PO, b.i.d. or t.i.d. Maximum, 4 mg daily in divided doses.

## Adverse reactions

Agitation • allergic rhinitis • *anxiety* • arthralgia • blurred vision • chest pain • *confusion* • *constipation* • *depression* • dermatitis • *diarrhea* • *difficulty speaking* • difficulty urinating • *dizziness* •

drowsiness • *dry mouth* • dysmenorrhea • dyspnea • hyperventilation • *fatigue* • *headache* • hot flushes • hypotension • *impaired coordination* • increased or decreased appetite • *insomnia* • *irritability* • lethargy • *lightheadedness* • malaise • mania • *memory impairment* • myalgia • nasal congestion • nausea • nervousness • palpitations • paresthesia • pruritus • *sedation* • sexual dysfunction • *somnolence* • sore throat • *suicide* • syncope • tremor • vertigo • vomiting

## Nursing considerations

■ Drug is contraindicated in patients with acute angle-closure glaucoma.

■ Use cautiously in patients with hepatic, renal, or pulmonary disease.

■ *Alert:* Don't withdraw drug abruptly; withdrawal symptoms, including seizures, may occur. Abuse or addiction is possible.

■ Monitor hepatic, renal, and hematopoietic function periodically in patients receiving repeated or prolonged therapy.

■ **Watch out!** Don't confuse alprazolam with alprostadil. Don't confuse Xanax with Zantac or Tenex.

22

# amiloride hydrochloride
(uh-MIL-uh-righd high-droh-KLOR-ighd)

Midamor

Pregnancy risk category: **B**

## Indications and dosages

**Hypertension; hypokalemia; edema from heart failure, usually in patients also taking thiazide or other potassium-wasting diuretics**
■ *Adults:* 5 mg P.O. daily, increased to 10 mg daily, if needed; then 15 mg. Maximum, 20 mg daily.
**Lithium-induced polyuria**
■ *Adults:* 10 to 20 mg P.O. daily.

## Adverse reactions

Abdominal pain ◦ *anorexia* ◦ **aplastic anemia** ◦ appetite changes ◦ constipation ◦ *diarrhea* ◦ dizziness ◦ dyspnea ◦ **encephalopathy** ◦ fatigue ◦ *headache* ◦ **hyperkalemia** ◦ hyponatremia ◦ impotence ◦ muscle cramps ◦ *nausea* ◦ **neutropenia** ◦ orthostatic hypotension ◦ *vomiting* ◦ weakness

## Nursing considerations

■ Drug is contraindicated in patients with potassium level higher than 5.5 mEq/L, anuria, acute or chronic renal insufficiency, or diabetic nephropathy.
■ Drug is contraindicated in patients receiving potassium supplementation or other potassium-sparing diuretics, such as spironolactone and triamterene.
■ Use cautiously in patients with diabetes mellitus, cardiopulmonary disease, or severe, existing hepatic or renal insufficiency.
■ Use cautiously in elderly or debilitated patients.
■ To prevent nausea, give drug with meals.
■ Monitor potassium level because of increased risk of hyperkalemia. Alert prescriber immediately if potassium level exceeds 5.5 mEq/L, and expect to stop drug.
■ Drug causes severe hyperkalemia in diabetic patients after glucose tolerance testing; stop drug at least 3 days before testing.
**Watch out!** Don't confuse amiloride with amiodarone.

# amiodarone hydrochloride

(am-ee-OH-dah-rohn high-dro-KLOR-ighd)

Cordarone, Pacerone

*Pregnancy risk category: D*

## Indications and dosages

**Life-threatening recurrent ventricular fibrillation or recurrent ventricular tachycardia unresponsive to adequate doses of other antiarrhythmics or when alternative drugs can't be tolerated**

■ *Adults:* Give loading dose of 800 to 1,600 mg P.O. daily divided b.i.d. for 1 to 3 weeks until first therapeutic response occurs; then 600 to 800 mg P.O. daily for 1 month, followed by maintenance dose of 200 to 600 mg P.O. daily. Or, give loading dose of 150 mg I.V. over 10 minutes (15 mg/minute); then 360 mg I.V. over next 6 hours (1 mg/ minute), followed by 540 mg I.V. over next 18 hours (0.5 mg/minute). After first 24 hours, continue with maintenance I.V. infusion of 720 mg/ 24 hours (0.5 mg/minute).

**Cardiac arrest, pulseless ventricular tachycardia, ventricular fibrillation**

■ *Adults:* 300 mg diluted in 20 to 30 ml of a compatible solution, as I.V. push.

**Supraventricular arrhythmias**

■ *Adults:* Give loading dose of 600 to 800 mg P.O. daily for 1 to 4 weeks or until supraventricular tachycardia is controlled or adverse reactions occur. Reduce gradually

---

to maintenance dose of 100 to 400 mg P.O. daily.

**Ventricular and supraventricular arrhythmias**

■ *Children:* Give loading dose of 10 to 15 mg/kg/day or 600 to 800 mg/1.73 m² P.O. daily for 4 to 14 days or until arrhythmia is controlled or adverse reactions occur. Reduce dosage to 5 mg/kg/day or 200 to 400 mg/1.73 m² for several weeks; then reduce dosage to lowest effective level. Or, give loading dose of 5 mg/kg I.V. infused over several minutes to 1 hour. Give additional 5-mg/kg loading dose if needed, to a maximum of 15 mg/kg/day. Or, 5 mg/kg I.V. in five divided doses of 1 mg/kg over 5 to 10 minutes to minimize exposure to diethylhexyl phthalate (DEHP).

**Short-term management of atrial fibrillation**

■ *Adults:* 125 mg/hour I.V. for 24 hours.

**Long-term management of recurrent atrial fibrillation**

■ *Adults:* 10 mg/kg P.O. daily for 14 days; then 300 mg P.O. daily for 4 weeks; then maintenance dosage of 200 mg P.O. daily.

**Heart failure (impaired ventricular ejection fraction, impaired exercise tolerance, and ventricular arrhythmias)**

■ *Adults:* 200 mg P.O. daily.

## amiodarone hydrochloride *(continued)*

### Adverse reactions

Abdominal pain • abnormal smell • abnormal taste • *acute respiratory distress syndrome* • anorexia • *arrhythmias* • asymptomatic corneal microdeposits • ataxia • blue-gray skin • *bradycardia* • *coagulation abnormalities* • constipation • edema • *fatigue* • headache • *heart block* • *heart failure* • hepatic dysfunction • *hepatic failure* • hyperthyroidism • hypotension • *hypothyroidism* • insomnia • *malaise* • *nausea* • optic neuropathy or neuritis resulting in visual impairment • paresthesia • peripheral neuropathy • *photosensitivity* • SEVERE PULMONARY TOXICITY • *sinus arrest* • sleep disturbances • solar dermatitis • *tremor* • *vision disturbances* • *vomiting*

### Nursing considerations

■ Drug is contraindicated in patients with cardiogenic shock, second- or third-degree antrioventricular block, or severe sinoatrial node disease resulting in bradycardia unless an artificial pacemaker is present and in those for whom bradycardia has caused syncope.

■ Give drug I.V. only where continuous ECG monitoring and electrophysiologic techniques are available. Mix first dose of 150 mg in 100 ml of $D_5W$ solution. Drug is incompatible with normal saline solution. When planning to give over 2 hours or longer, mix infusions in glass or polyolefin bottles.

■ Use an in-line filter with I.V. administration.

■ Whenever possible, give I.V. amiodarone through a central line dedicated to that purpose. If concentration is 2 mg/ml or more, use a central line.

■ Continuously monitor cardiac status of patient receiving drug I.V. If hypotension occurs, reduce infusion rate.

*Alert:* Cordarone I.V. leaches out plasticizers such as DEHP from I.V. tubing, which can adversely affect male reproductive tract development in fetuses, infants, and toddlers.

■ Be aware of the high risk of adverse reactions.

■ Obtain baseline pulmonary, liver, and thyroid function test results and baseline chest X-ray.

■ Give loading doses in a hospital setting and with continuous ECG monitoring because of the slow onset of antiarrhythmic effect and the risk of life-threatening arrhythmias.

■ Divide oral loading dose into two or three equal doses. Give maintenance dose once daily or divide into two doses. Give loading and maintenance doses with meals to decrease GI intolerance.

*(continued)*

*Alert:* Use only in patients with life-threatening, recurrent ventricular arrhythmias unresponsive to or intolerant of other antiarrhythmics or alternative drugs. Amiodarone can cause fatal toxicities, including hepatic and pulmonary toxicity.

*Alert:* Watch carefully for pulmonary toxicity. Risk increases in patients receiving doses over 400 mg/day. Monitor pulmonary function test results and chest X-ray.

▪ Monitor liver and thyroid function test results and electrolyte levels, particularly potassium and magnesium.

▪ Monitor PT and INR if patient takes warfarin and digoxin level if he takes digoxin.

▪ Instill methylcellulose ophthalmic solution during amiodarone therapy to minimize corneal microdeposits.

▪ Monitor blood pressure and heart rate and rhythm frequently. Perform continuous ECG monitoring when starting or changing dosage. Notify prescriber of significant change in assessment results.

▪ Life-threatening gasping syndrome may occur in neonates given I.V. solutions containing benzyl alcohol.

**Watch out!** Don't confuse amiodarone with amiloride.

# amitriptyline hydrochloride
(am-ih-TRIP-tuh-leen high-droh-KLOR-ighd)

Apo-Amitriptyline†

Pregnancy risk category: C

## Indications and dosages

**Depression**
■ *Adults:* Initially, 50 to 100 mg P.O. at bedtime, increasing to 150 mg daily. Maximum, 300 mg daily, if needed. Maintenance, 50 to 100 mg daily. Or, 20 to 30 mg I.M. q.i.d.
■ *Elderly patients and adolescents:* 10 mg P.O. t.i.d. and 20 mg P.O. at bedtime daily.

## Adverse reactions

*Agranulocytosis* • anorexia • anxiety • *arrhythmias* • ataxia • blurred vision • *coma* • constipation • delusions • diaphoresis • diarrhea • disorientation • dizziness • drowsiness • dry mouth • ECG changes • edema • eosinophilia • epigastric pain • extrapyramidal reactions • fatigue • hallucinations • headache • *heart block* • hyperglycemia • hypersensitivity reactions • hypertension • *hypoglycemia* • increased intraocular pressure • insomnia • *MI* • nausea • *orthostatic hypotension* • *leukopenia* • mydriasis • paralytic ileus • peripheral neuropathy • photosensitivity reactions • rash • restlessness • *seizures* • *stroke* • tachycardia • *thrombocytopenia* • tinnitus • tremor • urine retention • urticaria • vomiting • weakness

## Nursing considerations

■ Drug is contraindicated during acute recovery phase of MI and in patients who received an MAO inhibitor within past 14 days.
*Alert:* Parenteral form is for I.M. administration only. Drug shouldn't be given I.V.
■ Amitriptyline has strong anticholinergic effects and is one of the most sedating TCAs. Anticholinergic effects have rapid onset even though therapeutic effect is delayed for weeks.
■ Record mood changes. Monitor patient for suicidal tendencies and allow only minimum supply of drug.
■ Because patients using TCAs may suffer hypertensive episodes during surgery, stop drug gradually several days before planned surgery.
■ Monitor blood glucose level.
■ Don't withdraw drug abruptly.
**Watch out!** Don't confuse amitriptyline with nortriptyline or aminophylline.

# amlodipine besylate
(am-LOH-dih-peen BES-eh-layt)

Norvasc

Pregnancy risk category: C

## Indications and dosages

**Chronic stable angina, vaso-spastic angina (Prinzmetal's or variant angina)**
■ *Adults:* Initially, 5 to 10 mg P.O. daily. Most patients need 10 mg daily.
■ *Elderly patients:* Initially, 5 mg P.O. daily.
*Adjust-a-dose:* For patients who are small or frail or have hepatic insufficiency, initially 5 mg P.O. daily.

**Hypertension**
■ *Adults:* Initially, 2.5 to 5 mg P.O. daily. Dosage adjusted according to patient response and tolerance. Maximum dose, 10 mg daily.
■ *Elderly patients:* Initially, 2.5 mg P.O. daily.
*Adjust-a-dose:* For patients who are small or frail, are taking other antihypertensives, or have hepatic insufficiency, initially 2.5 mg P.O. daily.

## Adverse reactions

Abdominal pain • dizziness • dyspnea • *edema* • fatigue • flushing • headache • light-headedness • muscle pain • nausea • palpitations • paresthesia • pruritus • rash • sexual difficulties • somnolence

## Nursing considerations

*Alert:* Monitor patients carefully. Some patients, especially those with severe obstructive coronary artery disease, have developed increased frequency, duration, or severity of angina or acute MI after initiation of therapy with calcium channel blockers, such as amlodipine, or at time of dosage increase.
■ Monitor blood pressure frequently during initiation of therapy. Because drug-induced vasodilation has a gradual onset, acute hypotension is rare.
■ Notify prescriber if signs of heart failure, such as swelling of hands and feet or shortness of breath, occur.
**Watch out!** Don't confuse amlodipine with amiloride.

# amlodipine besylate and atorvastatin calcium
## (am-LOH-dih-peen BES-eh-layt and uh-TOR-vah-stah-tin KAL-see-um)

Caduet

Pregnancy risk category: X

## Indications and dosages

**Patients who need amlodipine for hypertension, chronic stable angina, or vasospastic angina and atorvastatin for heterozygous familial or nonfamilial hypercholesterolemia, mixed dyslipidemia, elevated serum triglyceride levels, primary dysbetalipoproteinemia, or homozygous familial hypercholesterolemia**

■ *Adults:* 5 to 10 mg amlodipine with 10 to 80 mg atorvastatin P.O. once daily. Determine the most effective dose for each component; then select the most appropriate combination product.

**Hypertension and heterozygous familial hypercholesterolemia in children**

■ *Boys and postmenarchal girls age 10 and older:* 5 mg amlodipine with 10 to 20 mg atorvastatin P.O. once daily. Determine the most effective dose for each component; then select the most appropriate combination product. If patient needs less than 5 mg of amlodipine, don't use the combination product.

## Adverse reactions

Abdominal pain ■ *allergic reaction* ■ *anaphylaxis* ■ arthralgia ■ arthritis ■ asthenia ■ back pain ■ bronchitis ■ chest pain ■ constipation ■ diarrhea ■ dizziness ■ dyspepsia ■ dyspnea ■ *edema* ■ fatigue ■ flatulence ■ flulike syndrome ■ flushing ■ *headache* ■ *infection* ■ insomnia ■ myalgia ■ nausea ■ palpitations ■ pharyngitis ■ pruritus ■ rash ■ rhinitis ■ sinusitis ■ somnolence ■ UTI ■ vertigo

## Nursing considerations

■ Use cautiously in patients who consume a lot of alcohol or have histories of hepatic disease.

■ Monitor liver function test results before therapy starts, after 12 weeks, whenever the dosage increases, and periodically during therapy.

■ Expect to reduce dose or stop drug if AST or ALT levels increase to more than 3 times the upper normal limit and remain elevated.

■ Assess patient for myalgia, muscle tenderness or weakness, and marked elevation in CK level. Expect to stop drug if CK level exceeds 10 times the upper normal limit or if myopathy is diagnosed.

■ Expect to stop drug if patient has a condition that increases the risk of renal failure secondary to rhabdomyolysis.

# amoxicillin and clavulanate potassium

(uh-moks-uh-SIL-in and
KLAV-yoo-lan-ayt poh-TAH-see-um)

Augmentin, Augmentin ES-600, Augmentin XR, Clavulin†

**Pregnancy risk category: B**

## Indications and dosages

▶ **Recurrent or persistent acute otitis media caused by Streptococcus pneumoniae, Haemophilus influenzae, or Moraxella catarrhalis in patients exposed to antibiotics within last 3 months who are age 2 or younger or are in day-care facilities**

■ *Children age 3 months and older:* 90 mg/kg/day Augmentin ES-600, PO, based on amoxicillin component, q 12 hours for 10 days.

▶ **Lower respiratory tract infections, otitis media, sinusitis, skin and skin-structure infections, and UTIs caused by susceptible strains of gram-positive and gram-negative organisms**

■ *Adults and children weighing 40 kg (88 lb) or more:* 250 mg PO, q 8 hours; or 500 mg PO, q 12 hours. For more severe infections, 500 mg PO, q 8 hours or 875 mg PO, q 12 hours.

■ *Children age 3 months and older weighing less than 40 kg:* 20 to 45 mg/kg PO, based on amoxicillin component and severity of infection, daily in divided doses q 8 to 12 hours.

■ *Children younger than age 3 months:* 30 mg/kg/day PO, based on amoxicillin component of the 125 mg/5-ml oral suspension, in divided doses q 12 hours.

**Adjust-a-dose:** Don't give the 875-mg tablet to patients with creatinine clearances less than 30 ml/minute. If clearance is 10 to 30 ml/minute, give 250 to 500 mg PO, q 12 hours. If clearance is less than 10 ml/minute, give 250 to 500 mg q 12 hours. For patients on hemodialysis, give 250 to 500 mg PO, q 24 hours with an additional dose during and after dialysis.

▶ **Community-acquired pneumonia or acute bacterial sinusitis caused by H. influenzae, M. catarrhalis, H. parainfluenzae, Klebsiella pneumoniae, methicillin-susceptible Staphylococcus aureus, or S. pneumoniae with reduced susceptibility to penicillin**

■ *Adults and children age 16 and older:* 2,000 mg/125 mg Augmentin XR tablets q 12 hours for 7 to 10 days for pneumonia; 10 days for sinusitis.

**Adjust-a-dose:** For patients with creatinine clearance less than 30 ml/minute and hemodialysis patients, don't use Augmentin XR.

## amoxicillin and clavulanate potassium
*(continued)*

### Adverse reactions

Abdominal pain • agitation • *agranulocytosis* • *anaphylaxis* • *angioedema* • anemia • anxiety • behavioral changes • black hairy tongue • confusion • *diarrhea* • dizziness • enterocolitis • eosinophilia • gastritis • glossitis • hypersensitivity reactions • indigestion • insomnia • *leukopenia* • mucocutaneous candidiasis • nausea • overgrowth of nonsusceptible organisms • pruritus • *pseudomembranous colitis* • rash • serum sickness–like reaction • stomatitis • *thrombocytopenia* • *thrombocytopenic purpura* • urticaria • vaginal candidiasis • vaginitis • vomiting

### Nursing considerations

■ Drug is contraindicated in patients with histories of amoxicillin-related cholestatic jaundice or hepatic dysfunction.

■ Drug is contraindicated in patients on hemodialysis and those with creatinine clearance less than 30 ml/minute.

■ Before giving drug, ask patient about allergic reactions to penicillin. However, a negative history of penicillin allergy is no guarantee against an allergic reaction.

■ Obtain specimen for culture and sensitivity testing before giving first dose. Therapy may begin pending results.

■ After reconstitution, refrigerate the oral suspension; discard after 10 days.

■ Give drug at least 1 hour before a bacteriostatic antibiotic.

■ Each Augmentin XR tablet contains 29.3 mg (1.27 mEq) of sodium.

■ Observe patient for signs and symptoms of superinfection.

*Alert:* Don't interchange the oral suspensions because of varying clavulanic acid contents.

■ Augmentin ES-600 is intended for children age 3 months to 12 years with persistent or recurrent acute otitis media only.

■ Avoid use of 250-mg tablet in children weighing less than 40 kg (88 lb). Give chewable form instead.

*Alert:* Both 250- and 500-mg film-coated tablets contain the same amount of clavulanic acid (125 mg). Therefore, two 250-mg tablets aren't equivalent to one 500-mg tablet. Regular tablets aren't equivalent to Augmentin XR.

**Watch out!** Don't confuse amoxicillin with amoxapine.

# amoxicillin trihydrate

(uh-moks-uh-trigh-HIGH-drayt)

Amoxil, Apo-Amoxi†, DisperMox†, Novamoxin†, Nu-Amoxi†, Trimox

**Pregnancy risk category:** B

## Indications and dosages

### Mild to moderate infections of the skin and skin structure, GU tract, or ear, nose, and throat

■ *Adults and children weighing 40 kg (88 lb) or more:* 500 mg PO. q 12 hours or 250 mg PO. q 8 hours.

■ *Children older than age 3 months weighing less than 40 kg:* 25 mg/kg/ day PO. divided q 12 hours or 20 mg/kg/day PO. divided q 8 hours.

■ *Neonates and infants up to age 3 months:* Up to 30 mg/kg/day PO. divided q 12 hours.

### Mild to severe infections of the lower respiratory tract and severe infections of the skin and skin structure, GU tract, or ear, nose, and throat

■ *Adults and children weighing 40 kg or more:* 875 mg PO. q 12 hours or 500 mg PO. q 8 hours.

■ *Children older than age 3 months weighing less than 40 kg:* 45 mg/kg/ day PO. divided q 12 hours or 40 mg/kg/day PO. divided q 8 hours.

### Uncomplicated gonorrhea

■ *Adults and children weighing more than 45 kg (99 lb):* 3 g PO. with 1 g probenecid given as a single dose.

■ *Children age 2 and older weighing less than 45 kg:* 50 mg/kg to a

maximum of 3 g PO. with 25 mg/kg to a maximum of 1 g of probenecid as a single dose. Don't give probenecid to children younger than age 2.

### To prevent endocarditis in patients having dental, oral, or respiratory tract procedures; for moderate-risk patients undergoing GI or GU procedures

■ *Adults:* 2 g PO. 1 hour before procedure.

■ *Children:* 50 mg/kg PO. 1 hour before procedure.

### To prevent penicillin-susceptible anthrax after exposure

■ *Adults and children older than age 9:* 500 mg PO. t.i.d. for 60 days.

■ *Children younger than age 9:* 80 mg/kg daily PO. divided t.i.d. for 60 days.

## Adverse reactions

Abdominal pain • agitation • **agranulocytosis** • **anaphylaxis** • anemia • anxiety • black hairy tongue • confusion • depression • **diarrhea** • dizziness • enterocolitis • eosinophilia • fatigue • gastritis • glossitis • hallucinations • hemolytic anemia • hypersensitivity reactions • interstitial nephritis • **leukopenia** • lethargy • **nausea** • nephropathy • overgrowth of nonsusceptible organisms • **pseudomembranous colitis** • **seizures** • stomatitis • **thrombocytopenia**

## amoxicillin trihydrate (continued)

* **thrombocytopenic purpura** *
vaginitis • vomiting

### Nursing considerations

■ Obtain specimen for culture and sensitivity testing before giving first dose. Therapy may begin pending results.

■ Before giving, ask patient about allergic reactions to penicillin. A negative history of penicillin allergy is no guarantee against allergic reaction.

■ Observe patient for signs and symptoms of superinfection.

■ Store Trimox oral suspension in refrigerator, if possible. It also may be stored at room temperature for up to 2 weeks.

**Watch out!** Don't confuse amoxicillin with amoxapine.

apomorphine hydrochloride

(uh-poh-MOR-feen high-droh-KLOR-ighd)

Apokyn

Pregnancy risk category: C

## Indications and dosages

■ **Intermittent hypomobility, "off" episodes caused by advanced Parkinson's disease**

*Adults:* Initially, give a 0.2-ml subQ test dose in a medically supervised setting. Measure supine and standing blood pressure q 20 minutes for the first hour. If patient tolerates and responds to drug, titrate dose starting with 0.2 ml subQ, p.r.n., as outpatient. Separate doses by at least 2 hours. Increase by 0.1 ml every few days, p.r.n. If initial 0.2-ml dose is ineffective but tolerated, give 0.4 ml subQ at next "off" period, measuring supine and standing blood pressure q 20 minutes for the first hour. If drug is tolerated, start with 0.3 ml subQ as outpatient. If needed, increase by 0.1 ml every few days. If patient doesn't tolerate 0.4-ml dose, give 0.3 ml subQ as test dose at next "off" period, measuring supine and standing blood pressure q 20 minutes for the first hour. If drug is tolerated, give 0.2 ml subQ as outpatient. Increase by 0.1 ml every few days, p.r.n. Doses higher than 0.4 ml usually aren't tolerated if 0.2 ml is the starting dose. Usual maximum dose is 0.6 ml subQ, p.r.n.

*Adjust-a-dose:* For patients with mild to moderate renal impairment, use test and starting doses of 0.1 ml subQ.

## Adverse reactions

*Angina* • aggravated Parkinson's disease • anxiety • arthralgia • back pain • bruising • **cardiac arrest** • *chest pain • chest pressure • confusion* • constipation • dehydration • depression • diarrhea • *dizziness* • *drowsiness* • dyskinesias • dyspnea • *edema • falls* • fatigue • flushing • hallucinations • headache • **heart failure** • *hypotension* • injection site reaction • insomnia • *limb pain • MI • nausea* • *orthostatic hypotension* • pallor • pneumonia • rhinorrhea • somnolence • sweating • syncope • UTI • *vomiting • weakness • yawning*

## Nursing considerations

■ **Alert:** Drug is for subQ injection only. Avoid I.V. use.

■ Give with an antiemetic to avoid severe nausea and vomiting. Start with trimethobenzamide 300 mg PO, t.i.d. 3 days before starting apomorphine, and continue antiemetic for at least 2 months.

■ **Alert:** The prescribed dosage should always be specified in milliliters rather than milligrams to avoid confusion; the dosing pen is marked in milliliters.

■ **Alert:** Monitor patient for drowsiness or sleepiness.

# aspirin (AS-prin)

Artria S.R., ASA, Aspergum, Bayer Aspirin, Coryphen†, Easprin, Ecotrin, Empirin, Entrophen†, Halfprin, Norwich Extra-Strength, Novasen†, ZORprin

Pregnancy risk category: D

## Indications and dosages

**Rheumatoid arthritis, osteoarthritis, other polyarthritic or inflammatory conditions**
■ *Adults:* Initially, 2.4 to 3.6 g P.O. daily in divided doses. Maintenance dosage, 3.2 to 6 g P.O. daily in divided doses.
**Juvenile rheumatoid arthritis**
■ *Children:* 60 to 110 mg/kg P.O. daily divided q 6 to 8 hours.
**Mild pain or fever**
■ *Adults and children older than age 11:* 325 to 650 mg P.O. or P.R. q 4 hours, p.r.n.
■ *Children ages 2 to 11:* 10 to 15 mg/kg/dose P.O. or P.R. q 4 hours up to 80 mg/kg daily.
**To prevent thrombosis**
■ *Adults:* 1.3 g P.O. in two to four divided doses.
**To reduce risk of MI in patients with previous MI or unstable angina**
■ *Adults:* 75 to 325 mg P.O. daily.
**Kawasaki syndrome**
■ *Adults:* 80 to 180 mg/kg P.O. daily in four divided doses during febrile phase. When fever subsides, decrease to 10 mg/kg once daily and adjust to salicylate level.
**Acute rheumatic fever**
■ *Adults:* 5 to 8 g P.O. daily.
■ *Children:* 100 mg/kg daily P.O. for 2 weeks; then 75 mg/kg daily P.O. for 4 to 6 weeks.

**To reduce risk of recurrent transient ischemic attacks and stroke or death in at-risk patients**
■ *Adults:* 50 to 325 mg P.O. daily.
**Acute ischemic stroke**
■ *Adults:* 160 to 325 mg P.O. daily, started within 48 hours of stroke onset and continued for up to 2 to 4 weeks.
**Acute pericarditis after MI**
■ *Adults:* 160 to 325 mg P.O. daily.

## Adverse reactions

*Angioedema* • bruising • dyspepsia • *GI bleeding* • hearing loss • *hepatitis* • hypersensitivity reactions • *leukopenia* • nausea • prolonged bleeding time • rash • *Reye's syndrome* • *thrombocytopenia* • tinnitus • urticaria

## Nursing considerations

■ Drug is contraindicated in patients with G6PD deficiency, bleeding disorders, or NSAID-induced sensitivity reactions.
■ Monitor salicylate level. Therapeutic salicylate level in arthritis is 150 to 300 mcg/ml.
■ Stop aspirin 5 to 7 days before elective surgery to allow time for production and release of new platelets.
**Watch out!** Don't confuse aspirin with Asendin or Afrin.

# atenolol (uh-TEN-uh-lol)

Apo-Atenolol[†], Tenormin

Pregnancy risk category: D

## Indications and dosages

### Hypertension
■ *Adults:* Initially, 50 mg P.O. daily alone or with a diuretic as a single dose, increased to 100 mg once daily after 7 to 14 days. Dosages of more than 100 mg daily are unlikely to produce further benefit.

### Angina pectoris
■ *Adults:* 50 mg P.O. once daily, increased, p.r.n., to 100 mg daily after 7 days for optimal effect. Maximum, 200 mg daily.

**To reduce risk of CV-related death and reinfarction in patients with acute MI**
■ *Adults:* 5 mg I.V. over 5 minutes; then another 5 mg after 10 minutes. After another 10 minutes, give 50 mg P.O., followed by another 50 mg P.O. in 12 hours. Subsequently, give 100 mg P.O. daily (as a single dose or 50 mg b.i.d.) for at least 7 days.

*Adjust-a-dose:* If creatinine clearance is 15 to 35 ml/minute, maximum dose is 50 mg daily; if clearance is less than 15 ml/minute, maximum dose is 25 mg daily. Hemodialysis patients need 25 to 50 mg after each dialysis session.

## Adverse reactions

***Bradycardia*** ■ ***bronchospasm*** ■ diarrhea ■ *dizziness* ■ drowsiness ■ dyspnea ■ *fatigue* ■ fever ■ ***heart failure*** ■ *hypotension* ■ intermittent claudication ■ leg pain ■ lethargy ■ nausea ■ rash ■ vertigo

## Nursing considerations

■ Drug is contraindicated in patients with sinus bradycardia, heart block (greater than first degree), overt cardiac failure, or cardiogenic shock.

■ Check apical pulse before giving drug; if it's slower than 60 beats/minute, withhold drug and call prescriber.

■ Monitor patient's blood pressure.

■ Monitor hemodialysis patients closely because of hypotension risk.

■ Beta-adrenergic blockers such as atenolol may mask tachycardia caused by hyperthyroidism. In patients with suspected thyrotoxicosis, expect to withdraw beta-adrenergic blocker gradually to avoid thyroid storm.

■ Drug may mask signs and symptoms of hypoglycemia in patients with diabetes.

*Alert:* Expect to withdraw drug gradually over 2 weeks to avoid serious adverse reactions.

**Watch out!** Don't confuse atenolol with albuterol or timolol.

# atorvastatin calcium
(uh-TOR-vah-stah-tin KAL-see-um)

Lipitor

Pregnancy risk category: X

## Indications and dosages

**Adjunct to diet to reduce LDL cholesterol, total cholesterol, apolipoprotein B, and triglyceride levels and to increase HDL cholesterol levels in patients with primary hypercholesterolemia (heterozygous familial and nonfamilial) and mixed dyslipidemia (Fredrickson types IIa and IIb); adjunct to diet to reduce triglyceride level (Fredrickson type IV); primary dysbetalipoproteinemia (Fredrickson type III) in patients who don't respond to diet**
■ *Adults:* Initially, 10 or 20 mg P.O. once daily. Patients who need a large reduction in LDL cholesterol (more than 45%) may be started at 40 mg once daily. Increase dosage, p.r.n., to maximum of 80 mg daily as a single dose. Dosage is based on lipid levels drawn within 2 to 4 weeks after starting therapy.
**To reduce total and LDL cholesterol in patients with homozygous familial hypercholesterolemia (alone or as an adjunct to lipid-lowering treatments such as LDL apheresis)**
■ *Adults:* 10 to 80 mg P.O. once daily.

**Heterozygous familial hyper-cholesterolemia**
■ *Children ages 10 to 17 (girls should be 1 year postmenarche):* Initially, 10 mg P.O. once daily. Adjustment intervals should be at least 4 weeks. Maximum dose, 20 mg daily.

## Adverse reactions

Abdominal pain ▪ allergic reactions ▪ arthralgia ▪ asthenia ▪ arthritis ▪ bronchitis ▪ constipation ▪ diarrhea ▪ dyspepsia ▪ flatulence ▪ flulike syndrome ▪ *headache* ▪ infection ▪ insomnia ▪ myalgia ▪ nausea ▪ peripheral edema ▪ pharyngitis ▪ rash ▪ rhinitis ▪ sinusitis ▪ UTI

## Nursing considerations

■ Drug is contraindicated in patients with active hepatic disease.
■ Use only after diet and other nondrug therapies prove ineffective. Patient should follow a standard low-cholesterol diet before and during therapy.
■ Obtain liver function tests and lipid levels before starting treatment, at 6 and 12 weeks after start of therapy, after an increase in dosage, and periodically thereafter.
■ Drug may be given as a single dose at any time of day, with or without food.
**Watch out!** Don't confuse Lipitor with Levatol.

# atropine sulfate (AH-troh-peen SUL-fayt)

Sal-Tropine

Pregnancy risk category: C

## Indications and dosages

**Symptomatic bradycardia, brady-arrhythmia (junctional or escape rhythm)**

- **Adults:** Usually, 0.5 to 1 mg I.V. push, repeated q 3 to 5 minutes to maximum of 2 mg, p.r.n.
- **Children and adolescents:** 0.02 mg/kg I.V., with minimum dose of 0.1 mg and maximum single dose of 0.5 mg in children and 1 mg in adolescents. May repeat dose at 5-minute intervals to a maximum total dose of 1 mg in children and 2 mg in adolescents.

**Antidote for anticholinesterase insecticide poisoning**

- **Adults:** Initially, 1 to 2 mg I.V.; may repeat with 2 mg I.M. or I.V. q 5 to 60 minutes until muscarinic signs and symptoms disappear or signs of atropine toxicity occur. Severe poisoning may require up to 6 mg hourly.
- **Children:** 0.05 mg/kg I.M. or I.V. repeated q 10 to 30 minutes until muscarinic signs and symptoms disappear (may be repeated if they reappear) or until signs of atropine toxicity occur.

**Preoperatively to diminish secretions and block cardiac vagal reflexes**

- **Adults and children weighing 20 kg (44 lb) or more:** 0.4 to 0.6 mg I.V., I.M., or SubQ 30 to 60 minutes before anesthesia.
- **Children weighing less than 20 kg:** 0.01 mg/kg I.V., I.M., or SubQ up to maximum dose of 0.4 mg 30 to 60 minutes before anesthesia. May repeat q 4 to 6 hours, p.r.n.
- **Infants weighing more than 5 kg (11 lb):** 0.03 mg/kg q 4 to 6 hours, p.r.n.
- **Infants weighing 5 kg or less:** 0.04 mg/kg q 4 to 6 hours, p.r.n.

**Adjunct treatment of peptic ulcer disease; functional GI disorders such as irritable bowel syndrome**

- **Adults:** 0.4 to 0.6 mg P.O. q 4 to 6 hours.

## Adverse reactions

Agitation • *anaphylaxis* • ataxia • *blurred vision* • **bradycardia** • confusion • *constipation* • cyclo-plegia • delirium • disorientation • dizziness • *dry mouth* • excitement • hallucinations • *headache* • impotence • increased intraocular pressure • *insomnia* • *mydriasis* • nausea • palpitations • photophobia • restlessness • *tachycardia* • thirst • urine retention • vomiting

## atropine sulfate *(continued)*

### Nursing considerations

■ Drug is contraindicated in patients with acute angle-closure glaucoma, obstructive uropathy, obstructive disease of the GI tract, paralytic ileus, toxic megacolon, intestinal atony, unstable CV status in acute hemorrhage, tachycardia, myocardial ischemia, asthma, or myasthenia gravis.

■ Use cautiously in patients with Down syndrome because they may be more sensitive to the drug.

■ Give I.V. into a large vein or into I.V. tubing over at least 1 minute.

■ Slow I.V. administration may cause paradoxical slowing of heart rate.

■ In adults, avoid doses less than 0.5 mg because of the risk of paradoxical bradycardia.

*Alert:* Watch for tachycardia in patients with cardiac conditions because it may lead to ventricular fibrillation.

# azithromycin (uh-zith-roh-MIGH-sin)

Zithromax

Pregnancy risk category: B

## Indications and dosages

**Acute bacterial worsening of COPD caused by *Haemophilus influenzae*, *Moraxella catarrhalis*, or *Streptococcus pneumoniae*; uncomplicated skin and skin-structure infections caused by *Staphylococcus aureus*, *Streptococcus pyogenes*, or *Streptococcus agalactiae*; second-line therapy for pharyngitis or tonsillitis caused by *S. pyogenes***

■ *Adults and adolescents age 16 and older:* Initially, 500 mg P.O. as a single dose on day 1, followed by 250 mg daily on days 2 through 5. Total cumulative dose, 1.5 g. Or, for worsening COPD, 500 mg P.O. daily for 3 days.

**Community-acquired pneumonia caused by *Chlamydia pneumoniae*, *H. influenzae*, *Mycoplasma pneumoniae*, *S. pneumoniae*, *Legionella pneumophila*, *M. catarrhalis*, or *S. aureus***

■ *Adults and adolescents age 16 and older:* For mild infections, 500 mg P.O. as a single dose on day 1; then 250 mg P.O. daily on days 2 through 5. Total dose, 1.5 g. For more severe infections or those caused by *S. aureus*, 500 mg I.V. as a single daily dose for 2 days; then 500 mg P.O. as a single daily dose to complete a 7- to 10-day course of therapy. Switch from I.V. to P.O. therapy based on patient response.

**Community-acquired pneumonia caused by *C. pneumoniae*, *H. influenzae*, *M. pneumoniae*, or *S. pneumoniae***

■ *Children age 6 months and older:* 10 mg/kg P.O. (maximum of 500 mg) as a single dose on day 1, followed by 5 mg/kg (maximum of 250 mg) daily on days 2 through 5.

**Chancroid**

■ *Adults:* 1 g P.O. as a single dose.

■ *Infants and children:* 20 mg/kg (maximum of 1 g) P.O. as a single dose.

**Nongonococcal urethritis or cervicitis caused by *Chlamydia trachomatis***

■ *Adults and adolescents age 16 and older:* 1 g P.O. as a single dose.

**Mycobacterium avium complex in patients with advanced HIV infection**

■ *Adults:* 600 mg P.O. daily with ethambutol 15 mg/kg daily.

**To prevent disseminated *M. avium* complex in patients with advanced HIV infection**

■ *Adults and adolescents:* 1.2 g P.O. once weekly alone or with rifabutin.

■ *Infants and children:* 20 mg/kg P.O. (maximum of 1.2 g) weekly or 5 mg/kg (maximum of 250 mg) P.O. daily. Children age 6 and older may also receive rifabutin 300 mg P.O. daily.

## azithromycin (continued)

**Urethritis and cervicitis caused by Neisseria gonorrhoeae**
■ *Adults:* 2 g P.O. as a single dose.

**Pelvic inflammatory disease caused by C. trachomatis, N. gonorrhoeae, or Mycoplasma hominis in patients who need initial I.V. therapy**
■ *Adults and adolescents age 16 and older:* 500 mg I.V. as a single daily dose for 1 to 2 days; then 250 mg P.O. daily to complete a 7-day course of therapy. Expect to switch from I.V. to P.O. therapy based on patient response.

**Otitis media**
■ *Children older than age 6 months:* 30 mg/kg P.O. as a single dose; or 10 mg/kg P.O. once daily for 3 days; or 10 mg/kg P.O. on day 1, then 5 mg/kg once daily on days 2 to 5.

**Pharyngitis, tonsillitis**
■ *Children age 2 and older:* 12 mg/kg (maximum of 500 mg) P.O. daily for 5 days.

**To prevent bacterial endocarditis in penicillin-allergic adults at moderate to high risk**
■ *Adults:* 500 mg P.O. 1 hour before procedure.
■ *Children:* 15 mg/kg P.O. 1 hour before procedure. Don't exceed adult dose.

**Chlamydial infections; uncomplicated gonococcal infections of the cervix, urethra, rectum, and pharynx; to prevent such infections after sexual assault**
■ *Adults:* 1 g P.O. as a single dose, with other drugs as recommended by the CDC.

### Adverse reactions

*Abdominal pain* ● **angioedema** ● candidiasis ● chest pain ● cholestatic jaundice ● *diarrhea* ● dizziness ● dyspepsia ● fatigue ● flatulence ● headache ● melena ● *nausea* ● nephritis ● palpitations ● photosensitivity ● **pseudomembranous colitis** ● rash ● somnolence ● vaginitis ● vertigo ● *vomiting*

### Nursing considerations

■ Drug is contraindicated in patients hypersensitive to erythromycin or other macrolides.
■ Obtain specimen for culture and sensitivity testing before giving first dose.
■ Infuse a 500-mg dose of azithromycin I.V. over 1 hour or longer.
■ Give multidose oral suspension 1 hour before or 2 hours after meals; don't give with antacids.
■ Monitor patient for signs and symptoms of superinfection.
■ Reconstitute single-dose, 1-g packets for suspension with 2 oz (60 ml) water; then mix and give to patient. Patient should rinse glass with additional 2 oz water and drink to ensure he has consumed entire dose. Packets aren't for pediatric use.

# benazepril hydrochloride
### (ben-AY-zuh-pril high-droh-KLOR-ighd)

Lotensin

*Pregnancy risk category: C; D in second and third trimesters*

## Indications and dosages

**Hypertension**
■ *Adults:* For patients not receiving a diuretic, 10 mg P.O. daily initially. Adjust dosage as needed and tolerated; usual dosage is 20 to 40 mg daily in one or two divided doses. For patients receiving a diuretic, 5 mg P.O. daily initially.
*Adjust-a-dose:* If creatinine clearance is below 30 ml/minute, give 5 mg P.O. daily. Daily dose may be adjusted up to 40 mg.

## Adverse reactions

Arthralgia ▪ arthritis ▪ dizziness ▪ drowsiness ▪ dry, persistent, non-productive cough ▪ fatigue ▪ headache ▪ **hyperkalemia** ▪ hypersensitivity reactions ▪ impotence ▪ increased diaphoresis ▪ myalgia ▪ nausea ▪ somnolence ▪ symptomatic hypotension

## Nursing considerations

■ Drug is contraindicated in patients hypersensitive to ACE inhibitors.
■ Monitor patient for hypotension. Excessive hypotension can occur when benazepril is given with diuretics.
■ Although ACE inhibitors such as benazepril reduce blood pressure in all races, they reduce it less in black patients taking the ACE inhibitor alone. Black patients should take drug with a thiazide diuretic for a more favorable response.
■ Drug may increase risk of angioedema in black patients.
■ Measure blood pressure when drug level is at peak (2 to 6 hours after administration) and at trough (just before a dose) to verify adequate blood pressure control.
■ Assess renal and hepatic function before and periodically during therapy. Monitor potassium level.
**Watch out!** Don't confuse benazepril with Benadryl. Don't confuse Lotensin with lovastatin or Loniten.

# bumetanide (byoo-MEH-tuh-nighd)

Bumex

Pregnancy risk category: C

## Indications and dosages

**Edema caused by heart failure or hepatic or renal disease**
■ *Adults:* 0.5 to 2 mg P.O. once daily. If diuretic response isn't adequate, a second or third dose may be given at 4- to 5-hour intervals. Maximum dosage, 10 mg daily. May be given parenterally if oral route isn't feasible. Usual first parenteral dose is 0.5 to 1 mg given I.V. or I.M. If response isn't adequate, a second or third dose may be given at 2- to 3-hour intervals. Maximum, 10 mg daily.

## Adverse reactions

Arthritic pain ▪ asymptomatic hyperuricemia ▪ azotemia ▪ chest pain ▪ diaphoresis ▪ diarrhea ▪ difficulty maintaining erection ▪ dizziness ▪ dry mouth ▪ ECG changes ▪ headache ▪ hypochloremic alkalosis ▪ hypokalemia ▪ hypomagnesemia ▪ muscle pain and tenderness ▪ nausea ▪ oliguria ▪ orthostatic hypotension ▪ pain ▪ premature ejaculation ▪ pruritus ▪ rash ▪ ***thrombocytopenia*** ▪ tinnitus ▪ transient deafness ▪ upset stomach ▪ vertigo ▪ volume depletion and dehydration ▪ vomiting ▪ *weakness*

## Nursing considerations

■ Drug is contraindicated in patients who are allergic to sulfonamides, in those with anuria or hepatic coma, and in those with severe electrolyte depletion.
■ Monitor fluid intake and output, weight, and electrolyte, BUN, creatinine, and carbon dioxide levels frequently.
■ Watch for evidence of hypokalemia, such as muscle weakness and cramps. Instruct patient to report these symptoms.
■ Consult prescriber and dietitian about a high-potassium diet. Foods rich in potassium include citrus fruits, tomatoes, bananas, dates, and apricots.
■ Monitor blood glucose level in patients with diabetes.
■ Monitor uric acid level, especially in patients with history of gout.
■ Monitor blood pressure and pulse rate during rapid diuresis.
■ Give I.V. doses over 1 to 2 minutes.
■ Bumetanide can be safely used in patients allergic to furosemide; 1 mg of bumetanide equals about 40 mg of furosemide.
**Watch out!** Don't confuse Bumex with Buprenex.

# bupropion hydrochloride
(byoo-PROH-pee-on high-droh-KLOR-ighd)

Wellbutrin, Wellbutrin SR, Wellbutrin XL

Pregnancy risk category: B

## Indications and dosages

**Depression**

■ *Adults:* For immediate-release form, initially, 100 mg P.O. b.i.d.; increase after 3 days to 100 mg P.O. t.i.d., if needed. If patient doesn't improve after several weeks of therapy, increase dosage to 150 mg t.i.d. No single dose should exceed 150 mg. Allow at least 6 hours between successive doses. Maximum, 450 mg daily. For sustained-release form, initially, 150 mg P.O. q morning; increase to target dosage of 150 mg P.O. b.i.d., as tolerated, as early as day 4 of dosing. Allow at least 8 hours between successive doses. Maximum, 400 mg daily. For extended-release form, initially, 150 mg P.O. q morning; increase to target dosage of 300 mg P.O. daily, as tolerated, as early as day 4 of dosing. Allow at least 24 hours between successive doses. Maximum, 450 mg daily.

**Adjust-a-dose:** For patients with mild to moderate hepatic cirrhosis or renal impairment, reduce frequency and dosage. For patients with severe hepatic cirrhosis, don't exceed 75 mg (immediate-release) P.O. daily, 100 mg (sustained-release) P.O. daily, 150 mg (sustained-release or extended-release) P.O. every other day.

## Nursing considerations

■ Drug is contraindicated in patients who have taken MAO inhibitors within previous 14 days and in those with seizure disorders or history of bulimia or anorexia nervosa.

*Alert:* Carefully monitor patient for worsening depression or suicidal thoughts.

**Watch out!** Don't confuse bupropion with buspirone. Don't confuse Wellbutrin with Wellcovorin.

## Adverse reactions

Abdominal pain • agitation • akathisia • akinesia • anorexia • anxiety • **arrhythmias** • arthralgia • auditory disturbances • blurred vision • chest pain • confusion • constipation • decreased libido • delusions • diarrhea • dizziness • *dry mouth* • dyspepsia • epistaxis • euphoria • *excessive diaphoresis* • fatigue • fever • *headache* • hypertension • hypotension • impotence • increased appetite • *insomnia* • menstrual complaints • muscle spasm • *nausea* • palpitations • *pharyngitis* • pruritus • rash • sedation • **seizures** • **suicidal behavior** • sinusitis • syncope • *tachycardia* • taste disturbance • tremor • urinary frequency • urine retention • vomiting • *weight gain or loss*

## captopril (KAP-toh-pril)

*Capoten, Novo-Captoril†*

Pregnancy risk category: C; D in second and third trimesters

### Indications and dosages

**Hypertension**

■ *Adults:* Initially, 25 mg P.O. b.i.d. or t.i.d. If blood pressure isn't controlled satisfactorily in 1 or 2 weeks, increase dosage to 50 mg b.i.d. or t.i.d. If that dosage doesn't control blood pressure satisfactorily after another 1 or 2 weeks, expect to add a diuretic. If patient needs further blood pressure reduction, dosage may be raised to 150 mg t.i.d. while continuing diuretic. Maximum dosage, 450 mg daily.

**Diabetic nephropathy**

■ *Adults:* 25 mg P.O. t.i.d.

**Heart failure**

■ *Adults:* Initially, 25 mg P.O. t.i.d. Patients with normal or low blood pressure who have been vigorously treated with diuretics and who may be hyponatremic or hypovolemic may start with 6.25 or 12.5 mg P.O. t.i.d.; starting dosage may be adjusted over several days. Gradually increase dosage to 50 mg P.O. t.i.d.; delay further dosage increases for at least 2 weeks. Maximum dosage, 450 mg daily.

■ *Elderly patients:* Initially, 6.25 mg P.O. b.i.d. Increase gradually, p.r.n.

**Left ventricular dysfunction after acute MI**

■ *Adults:* Start therapy as early as 3 days after MI with 6.25 mg P.O.

for one dose, followed by 12.5 mg P.O. t.i.d. Increase over several days to 25 mg P.O. t.i.d.; then increase to 50 mg P.O. t.i.d. over several weeks.

### Adverse reactions

Abdominal pain ▪ *agranulocytosis* ▪ alopecia ▪ anemia ▪ *angioedema* ▪ angina pectoris ▪ anorexia ▪ constipation ▪ diarrhea ▪ dizziness ▪ dry mouth ▪ *dry, persistent, nonproductive cough* ▪ dysgeusia ▪ dyspnea ▪ fainting ▪ fatigue ▪ fever ▪ headache ▪ hyperkalemia ▪ hypotension ▪ *leukopenia* ▪ maculopapular rash ▪ malaise ▪ nausea ▪ *pancytopenia* ▪ pruritus ▪ tachycardia ▪ *thrombocytopenia* ▪ urticarial rash ▪ vomiting

### Nursing considerations

■ Monitor patient's blood pressure and pulse rate frequently.

*Alert:* Elderly patients may be more sensitive to drug's hypotensive effects.

■ In patients with impaired renal function or collagen vascular disease, monitor WBC and differential counts before starting treatment, every 2 weeks for the first 3 months of therapy, and periodically thereafter.

**Watch out!** Don't confuse captopril with Capitrol.

# carvedilol (kar-VAY-deh-lol)

Coreg

Pregnancy risk category: C

## Indications and dosages

**Hypertension**

■ *Adults:* Dosage highly individualized. Initially, 6.25 mg P.O. b.i.d. Measure standing blood pressure 1 hour after first dose. If tolerated, continue dosage for 7 to 14 days. May increase to 12.5 mg P.O. b.i.d. for 7 to 14 days, following same blood pressure monitoring protocol as before. Maximum dosage, 25 mg P.O. b.i.d., as tolerated.

**Left ventricular dysfunction after MI**

■ *Adults:* Dosage individualized. Start therapy after patient is hemodynamically stable and fluid retention has been minimized. Initially, 6.25 mg P.O. b.i.d. Increase after 3 to 10 days to 12.5 mg b.i.d., then again to a target dosage of 25 mg b.i.d. Or, start with 3.25 mg b.i.d.; or adjust dosage more slowly if indicated.

**Mild to severe heart failure**

■ *Adults:* Dosage highly individualized. Initially, 3.125 mg P.O. b.i.d. for 2 weeks; if tolerated, may increase to 6.25 mg P.O. b.i.d. Dosage may be doubled q 2 weeks as tolerated. Maximum dosage for patients weighing more than 85 kg (187 lb) is 50 mg P.O. b.i.d. For patients weighing less than 85 kg, maximum dosage is 25 mg P.O. b.i.d.

*Adjust-a-dose:* Use reduced dosage if patient's pulse rate is below 55 beats/minute.

**Angina pectoris**

■ *Adults:* 25 to 50 mg P.O. b.i.d.

**Idiopathic cardiomyopathy**

■ *Adults:* 6.25 to 25 mg P.O. b.i.d.

## Adverse reactions

Abdominal pain • abnormal renal function • abnormal vision • albuminuria • anemia • angina • arthralgia • *asthenia* • **AV block** • back pain • blurred vision • **brady-cardia** • bronchitis • chest pain • cough • depression • *diarrhea* • *dizziness* • dyspepsia • dyspnea • edema • *fatigue* • fever • flulike syndrome • glycosuria • headache • hematuria • fluid overload • gout • hypercholesterolemia • *hyper-glycemia* • **hyperkalemia** • *hyper-sensitivity reactions* • hypertri-glyceridemia • hyperuricemia • hypoesthesia • hypertension • **hypoglycemia** • hyponatremia • *hypotension* • hypotonia • hypo-volemia • infection • impotence • insomnia • **lung edema** • malaise • melena • muscle cramps • nau-sea • pain • palpitations • pares-thesia • periodontitis • peripheral edema • peripheral vascular dis-order • pharyngitis • purpura • rhinitis • sinusitis • somnolence • **stroke** • syncope • **thrombocy-topenia** • vertigo • vomiting • *weight gain* • weight loss

## carvedilol *(continued)*

### Nursing considerations

■ Drug is contraindicated in patients with New York Heart Association class IV decompensated cardiac failure requiring inotropic therapy, bronchial asthma or related conditions, second- or third-degree heart block, sick sinus syndrome (unless a pacemaker is in place), cardiogenic shock, or severe bradycardia.

*Alert:* Patients receiving therapy with beta-adrenergic blockers such as carvedilol who have a history of severe anaphylactic reaction to several allergens may be more reactive to repeated challenge (accidental, diagnostic, or therapeutic). They may be unresponsive to dosages of epinephrine typically used to treat allergic reactions.

■ If drug must be stopped, do so gradually over 1 to 2 weeks.

■ Monitor patient with heart failure for worsened condition, renal dysfunction, or fluid retention; diuretic dosage may need to be increased.

■ Monitor patient with diabetes closely; drug may mask signs and symptoms of hypoglycemia, or hyperglycemia may worsen.

■ Observe patient for dizziness or light-headedness for 1 hour after giving each new dose.

■ Monitor elderly patients carefully; drug levels are about 50% higher in elderly patients than in younger patients.

# cefazolin sodium (sef-EH-zoh-lin SOH-dee-um)

Ancet

Pregnancy risk category: B

## Indications and dosages

**Perioperative prevention in contaminated surgery**

■ *Adults:* 1 g I.M. or I.V. 30 to 60 minutes before surgery; then 0.5 to 1 g I.M. or I.V. q 6 to 8 hours for 24 hours. In operations lasting longer than 2 hours, give another 0.5- to 1-g dose I.M. or I.V. intraoperative-ly. Continue treatment for 3 to 5 days if life-threatening infection is likely.

**Infections of respiratory, biliary, and GU tracts; skin, soft-tissue, bone, and joint infections; septicemia; endocarditis caused by *Escherichia coli, Enterobacteriaceae* organisms; gonococci, *Haemophilus influenzae, Klebsiella* species, *Proteus mirabilis, Staphylococcus aureus, Streptococcus pneumoniae,* and group A beta-hemolytic streptococci**

■ *Adults:* 250 to 500 mg I.M. or I.V. q 8 hours for mild infections, or 500 mg to 1.5 g I.M. or I.V. q 6 to 8 hours for moderate to severe or life-threatening infections. Maximum dosage, 12 g/day in life-threatening situations.

■ *Children older than age 1 month:* 25 to 50 mg/kg/day I.M. or I.V. in three or four divided doses. In severe infections, may increase dose to 100 mg/kg/day.

**Adjust-a-dose:** For patients with creatinine clearance of 35 to 54 ml/minute, give full dose q 8 hours. If clearance is 11 to 34 ml/minute, give 50% usual dose q 12 hours. If clearance is below 10 ml/minute, give 50% of usual dose q 18 to 24 hours.

## Adverse reactions

Abdominal cramps • anal pruritus • anaphylaxis • anorexia • candidiasis • confusion • diarrhea • drug fever • dyspepsia • eosinophilia • genital pruritus • glossitis • headache • hypersensitivity reactions • induration • leukopenia • maculopapular and erythematous rash • nausea • neutropenia • oral candidiasis • pain • phlebitis • pruritus • pseudomembranous colitis • seizures • serum sickness • sterile abscesses • Stevens-Johnson syndrome • thrombophlebitis (with I.V. injection) • thrombocytopenia • tissue sloughing at injection site • urticaria • vaginitis • vomiting

## Nursing considerations

■ Before administration, ask patient if he's allergic to penicillins or cephalosporins.

## cefazolin sodium *(continued)*

■ Reconstitute drug with sterile water for injection, bacteriostatic water, or normal saline solution as follows: Add 2 ml to 500-mg vial or 2.5 ml to 1-g vial, yielding 225 mg/ml or 330 mg/ml, respectively. Shake well until dissolved.

■ Reconstituted drug is stable for 24 hours at room temperature or 96 hours under refrigeration.

■ For direct injection, further dilute with 5 ml of sterile water for injection. Inject into a large vein or into the tubing of a free-flowing I.V. solution over 3 to 5 minutes. For intermittent infusion, add reconstituted drug to 50 to 100 ml of compatible solution or use premixed solution. Give commercially available frozen solutions of cefazolin in $D_5W$ only by intermittent or continuous I.V. infusion.

■ Alternate injection sites if I.V. therapy lasts longer than 3 days. Use of small I.V. needles in larger available veins may be preferable.

■ Obtain specimen for culture and sensitivity testing before giving first dose. Therapy may begin pending results.

■ After reconstitution, inject drug I.M. Give injection deeply into a large muscle such as the gluteus maximus.

■ Monitor patient for signs and symptoms of superinfection.

**Watch out!** Don't confuse cefazolin with other cephalosporins that sound alike.

## cefepime hydrochloride
(sef-eh-PIME high-droh-KLOR-ighd)

Maxipime

Pregnancy risk category: B

### Indications and dosages

**Mild to moderate UTIs caused by *Escherichia coli, Klebsiella pneumoniae,* or *Proteus mirabilis,* including concurrent bacteremia with these microorganisms**

■ *Adults and children age 12 and older:* 0.5 to 1 g I.M. or I.V. infused over 30 minutes q 12 hours for 7 to 10 days. I.M. route used only for *E. coli* infections.

**Severe UTIs, including pyelonephritis, caused by *E. coli* or *K. pneumoniae***

■ *Adults and children age 12 and older:* 2 g I.V. infused over 30 minutes q 12 hours for 10 days.

**Moderate to severe pneumonia caused by *Streptococcus pneumoniae, Pseudomonas aeruginosa, K. pneumoniae,* or *Enterobacter* species**

■ *Adults and children age 12 and older:* 1 to 2 g I.V. infused over 30 minutes q 12 hours for 10 days.

**Moderate to severe skin infections, uncomplicated skin infections, and skin-structure infections caused by *Streptococcus pyogenes* or methicillin-susceptible strains of *Staphylococcus aureus***

■ *Adults and children age 12 and older:* 2 g I.V. infused over 30 minutes q 12 hours for 10 days.

**Complicated intra-abdominal infections caused by *E. coli,* viridans group streptococci, *P. aeruginosa, K. pneumoniae, Enterobacter* species, or *Bacteroides fragilis***

■ *Adults:* 2 g I.V. infused over 30 minutes q 12 hours for 7 to 10 days. Use with metronidazole.

**Empiric therapy for febrile neutropenia**

■ *Adults:* 2 g I.V. q 8 hours for 7 days or until neutropenia resolves.

**Uncomplicated and complicated UTIs (including pyelonephritis), uncomplicated skin and skin-structure infections, pneumonia in children; as empiric therapy for febrile neutropenic children**

■ *Children ages 2 months to 16 years weighing up to 40 kg (88 lb):* 50 mg/kg/dose I.V. infused over 30 minutes q 12 hours (q 8 hours for febrile neutropenia) for 7 to 10 days. Don't exceed 2 g/dose.

*Adjust-a-dose:* Reduce dose for patients with renal impairment. For patients receiving hemodialysis, about 68% of drug is removed after a 3-hour dialysis session. Give a repeat dose, equivalent to the first dose, at the completion of dialysis. For patients receiving continuous ambulatory peritoneal dialysis, give normal dosage q 48 hours.

## cefepime hydrochloride *(continued)*

### Adverse reactions

**Anaphylaxis** • colitis • diarrhea • fever • headache • hypersensitivity reactions • inflammation • nausea • oral candidiasis • pain • phlebitis • pruritus • rash • urticaria • vaginitis • vomiting

### Nursing considerations

■ Before administration, ask patient if he's allergic to penicillins or cephalosporins.

■ Obtain specimen for culture and sensitivity testing before giving first dose. Therapy may begin pending results.

■ For I.M. administration, reconstitute according to manufacturer's guidelines.

■ Inspect solution for particulate matter before use; powder and its solutions tend to darken.

■ Monitor patient for signs and symptoms of superinfection.

■ Monitor PT and INR in patients requiring prolonged therapy, as ordered. Give exogenous vitamin K, as indicated.

**Watch out!** Don't confuse cefepime with other cephalosporins that sound alike.

## ceftazidime (sef-TAZ-ih-deem)

Ceptaz, Fortaz, Tazicef, Tazidime

Pregnancy risk category: B

### Indications and dosages

**Serious UTIs and lower respiratory tract infections; skin, gynecologic, intra-abdominal, and CNS infections; bacteremia; and septicemia caused by susceptible microorganisms, such as streptococci, penicillinase- and non-penicillinase-producing *Staphylococcus aureus*, *Escherichia coli*, *Klebsiella* species, *Proteus* species, *Enterobacter* species, *Haemophilus influenzae*, *Pseudomonas* species, and some strains of *Bacteroides***

■ *Adults and children age 12 and older:* 1 to 2 g I.V. or I.M. q 8 to 12 hours; up to 6 g daily in life-threatening infections.

■ *Children ages 1 month to 11 years:* 25 to 50 mg/kg I.V. q 8 hours. Maximum dosage, 6 g/day. Use sodium carbonate formulation.

■ *Neonates up to age 4 weeks:* 30 mg/kg I.V. q 12 hours. Use sodium carbonate formulation.

**Uncomplicated UTIs**

■ *Adults:* 250 mg I.V. or I.M. q 12 hours.

**Complicated UTIs**

■ *Adults and children age 12 and older:* 500 mg to 1 g I.V. or I.M. q 8 to 12 hours.

*Adjust-a-dose:* For renally impaired patients, if creatinine clearance is 31 to 50 ml/minute, give 1 g q 12 hours;

if clearance is 16 to 30 ml/minute, give 1 g q 24 hours; if clearance is 6 to 15 ml/ minute, give 500 mg q 24 hours; if clearance is less than 5 ml/ minute, give 500 mg q 48 hours. Because ceftazidime is removed by hemodialysis, give a dose of drug after each dialysis treatment.

### Adverse reactions

Abdominal cramps • *agranulocytosis* • *anaphylaxis* • candidiasis • diarrhea • dizziness • eosinophilia • headache • hemolytic anemia • hypersensitivity reactions • *induration* • *leukopenia* • nausea • *pain* • paresthesia • *phlebitis* • *pseudomembranous colitis* • rash • *seizures* • serum sickness • sterile abscesses • *thrombocytopenia* • thrombocytosis • thrombophlebitis • tissue sloughing at injection site • urticaria • vaginitis • vomiting

### Nursing considerations

■ Before administration, ask patient if he's allergic to penicillins or cephalosporins.

■ Infuse drug over 15 to 30 minutes.

■ For I.M. administration, inject deeply into a large muscle such as the gluteus maximus.

**Watch out!** Don't confuse ceftazidime with other cephalosporins that sound alike.

## celecoxib (sel-eh-COKS-ib)

Celebrex

Pregnancy risk category: C; D in third trimester

### Indications and dosages

**Relief from signs and symptoms of osteoarthritis**
■ *Adults:* 200 mg P.O. daily as a single dose or divided equally b.i.d.
**Relief from signs and symptoms of rheumatoid arthritis**
■ *Adults:* 100 to 200 mg P.O. b.i.d.
**Adjunctive treatment for familial adenomatous polyposis to reduce the number of adenomatous colorectal polyps**
■ *Adults:* 400 mg P.O. b.i.d. with food for up to 6 months.
■ *Elderly patients:* Start at lowest dosage.
**Acute pain and primary dysmenorrhea**
■ *Adults:* Initially, 400 mg P.O., followed by an additional 200-mg dose if needed. On subsequent days, 200 mg P.O. b.i.d., p.r.n.
■ *Elderly patients:* Start at lowest dosage.
*Adjust-a-dose:* For patients weighing less than 50 kg (110 lb), start at lowest dosage. For patients with Child-Pugh class II hepatic impairment, start with reduced dosage.

### Adverse reactions

Abdominal pain • accidental injury • back pain • diarrhea • dizziness • dyspepsia • flatulence • *headache* • hyperchloremia • insomnia • nausea • peripheral edema • pharyngitis • rash • rhinitis • sinusitis • upper respiratory tract infection

### Nursing considerations

■ Drug is contraindicated in patients hypersensitive to sulfonamides, aspirin, or other NSAIDs and in those with severe hepatic or renal impairment.
*Alert:* Patients may be allergic to drug if they're allergic to or have had anaphylactic reactions to sulfonamides, aspirin, or other NSAIDs.
■ Drug can be given without regard to meals, but food may decrease GI upset.
■ Watch for signs and symptoms of overt and occult bleeding.
■ NSAIDs such as celecoxib can cause fluid retention; monitor patient with hypertension, edema, or heart failure.
■ Watch for signs and symptoms of hepatotoxicity.
■ Before starting drug therapy, rehydrate dehydrated patient.
**Watch out!** Don't confuse Celebrex with Cerebyx or Celexa.

## cephalexin (sef-uh-LEK-sin)

cephalexin hydrochloride
**Keftab**
cephalexin monohydrate
**Apo-Cephalex†, Biocef, Keflex, Novo-Lexin†, Nu-Cephalex†**

Pregnancy risk category: **B**

### Indications and dosages

**Respiratory tract, GI tract, skin, soft-tissue, bone, and joint infections and otitis media caused by** *Escherichia coli* **and other coliform bacteria, group A beta-hemolytic streptococci,** *Klebsiella* **species,** *Proteus mirabilis, Streptococcus pneumoniae,* **and staphylococci**

■ *Adults:* 250 mg to 1 g P.O. q 6 hours, or 500 mg q 12 hours. Maximum dosage, 4 g daily.
■ *Children:* 25 to 50 mg/kg/day P.O. in two to four equally divided doses. In severe infections, dose can be doubled.
*Adjust-a-dose:* For adults with impaired renal function, initial dose is the same. For subsequent dosing in patients with creatinine clearance less than 5 ml/minute, give 250 mg P.O. q 12 to 24 hours; for clearance of 5 to 10 ml/minute, give 250 mg P.O. q 12 hours; and for clearance of 11 to 40 ml/minute, give 500 mg P.O. q 8 to 12 hours.

### Adverse reactions

Abdominal pain ▪ agitation ▪ anal pruritus ▪ **anaphylaxis** ▪ anemia ▪ *anorexia* ▪ arthralgia ▪ arthritis ▪ candidiasis ▪ confusion ▪ *diarrhea* ▪ dizziness ▪ dyspepsia ▪ eosinophilia ▪ fatigue ▪ gastritis ▪ genital pruritus ▪ glossitis ▪ hallucinations ▪ headache ▪ hypersensitivity reactions ▪ interstitial nephritis ▪ joint pain ▪ *maculopapular and erythematous rashes* ▪ nausea ▪ **neutropenia** ▪ oral candidiasis ▪ **pseudomembranous colitis** ▪ serum sickness ▪ tenesmus ▪ **thrombocytopenia** ▪ urticaria ▪ vaginitis ▪ vomiting

### Nursing considerations

■ Ask patient about past reaction to cephalosporin or penicillin therapy before giving first dose.
■ Obtain specimen for culture and sensitivity testing before giving first dose.
■ To prepare oral suspension: Add required amount of water to powder in two portions. Shake well after each addition. After mixing, store in refrigerator. Mixture will remain stable for 14 days. Keep tightly closed and shake well before using.
■ Monitor patient for signs and symptoms of superinfection.
■ Treat group A beta-hemolytic streptococcal infections for a minimum of 10 days.
**Watch out!** Don't confuse cephalexin with other cephalosporins that sound alike.

## cetirizine hydrochloride
(seh-TEER-ih-zeen high-droh-KLOR-ighd)

Zyrtec

Pregnancy risk category: B

## Indications and dosages

**Seasonal allergic rhinitis**
■ *Adults and children age 6 and older:* 5 to 10 mg P.O. once daily.
■ *Children ages 2 to 5:* 2.5 mg P.O. once daily. Maximum dosage, 5 mg daily.

**Perennial allergic rhinitis, chronic urticaria**
■ *Adults and children age 6 and older:* 5 to 10 mg P.O. once daily.
■ *Children ages 6 months to 5 years:* 2.5 mg P.O. once daily; in children ages 1 to 5, increase to maximum of 5 mg daily in two divided doses.
*Adjust-a-dose:* For adults and children ages 6 and older receiving hemodialysis, those with hepatic impairment, and those with creatinine clearance less than 31 ml/minute, give 5 mg P.O. daily. Don't use in children younger than age 6 with renal or hepatic impairment.

## Adverse reactions

Abdominal distress • dizziness • dry mouth • fatigue • headache • nausea • pharyngitis • *somnolence* • vomiting

## Nursing considerations

■ Drug is contraindicated in patients hypersensitive to hydroxyzine.
■ Stop drug 4 days before diagnostic skin testing because antihistamines can prevent, reduce, or mask positive skin test response.
**Watch out!** Don't confuse Zyrtec with Zantac or Zyprexa.

# ciprofloxacin (sih-proh-FLOKS-uh-sin)

Cipro, Cipro I.V. Cipro XR

Pregnancy risk category: C

## Indications and dosages

**Mild to moderate UTIs caused by Escherichia coli, Klebsiella pneumoniae, Enterobacter cloacae, Serratia marcescens, Proteus mirabilis, Providencia rettgeri, Morganella morganii, Citrobacter diversus, Citrobacter freundii, Pseudomonas aeruginosa, Staphylococcus epidermidis, and Enterococcus faecalis**
- *Adults:* 250 mg P.O. or 200 mg I.V. q 12 hours.

**Severe or complicated UTIs; mild to moderate bone and joint infections caused by E. cloacae, P. aeruginosa, and S. marcescens; mild to moderate respiratory infections caused by E. coli, K. pneumoniae, E. cloacae, P. mirabilis, P. aeruginosa, Haemophilus influenzae, and Haemophilus parainfluenzae; mild to moderate skin and skin-structure infections caused by E. coli, K. pneumoniae, E. cloacae, P. mirabilis, P. vulgaris, Providencia stuartii, M. morganii, C. freundii, Streptococcus pyogenes, P. aeruginosa, Staphylococcus aureus, and S. epidermidis; infectious diarrhea caused by E. coli, Campylobacter jejuni, Shigella flexneri, and Shigella sonnei; typhoid fever**
- *Adults:* 500 mg P.O. or 400 mg I.V. q 12 hours.

**Severe or complicated bone or joint infections, severe respiratory tract infections, severe skin and skin-structure infections**
- *Adults:* 750 mg P.O. q 12 hours, or 400 mg I.V. q 8 to 12 hours.

**Chronic bacterial prostatitis caused by E. coli or P. mirabilis**
- *Adults:* 500 mg P.O. q 12 hours or 400 mg I.V. q 12 hours for 28 days.

**Complicated intra-abdominal infections caused by E. coli, P. aeruginosa, P. mirabilis, K. pneumoniae, or Bacteroides fragilis**
- *Adults:* 500 mg P.O. or 400 mg I.V. q 12 hours for 7 to 14 days. Give with metronidazole.

**Acute uncomplicated cystitis**
- *Adults:* 100 mg or 250 mg P.O. q 12 hours for 3 days.

**Uncomplicated UTIs**
- *Adults:* 500 mg extended-release tablet P.O. once daily for 3 days.

**Mild to moderate acute sinusitis caused by H. influenzae, Streptococcus pneumoniae, or Moraxella catarrhalis**
- *Adults:* 500 mg P.O. or 400 mg I.V. q 12 hours for 10 days.

56

## ciprofloxacin *(continued)*

**Empirical therapy in febrile neu-
tropenic patients**

■ *Adults:* 400 mg I.V. q 8 hours
used with piperacillin 50 mg/kg I.V.
q 4 hours (not to exceed 24 g/day).

**Inhalation anthrax (postexposure)**

■ *Adults:* Initially, 400 mg I.V. q 12
hours until susceptibility test results
are known; then 500 mg P.O. b.i.d.

■ *Children:* 10 mg/kg I.V. q 12 hours;
then 15 mg/kg P.O. q 12 hours.
Don't exceed 800 mg/day I.V. or
1,000 mg/day P.O.

■ *For all patients:* Give drug with
one or two additional antimicro-
bials. Switch to oral therapy when
appropriate. Treat for 60 days (I.V.
and P.O. combined).

**Cutaneous anthrax**

■ *Adults:* 500 mg P.O. b.i.d. for 60
days.

■ *Children:* 10 to 15 mg/kg q 12
hours. Don't exceed 1,000 mg/day.
Treat for 60 days.

*Adjust-a-dose:* For patients with
creatinine clearance of 30 to 50 ml/
minute, give 250 to 500 mg P.O.
q 12 hours or the usual I.V. dose. If
clearance is 5 to 29 ml/minute, give
250 to 500 mg P.O. q 18 hours or
200 to 400 mg I.V. q 18 to 24 hours.
If patient is receiving hemodialysis,
give 250 to 500 mg P.O. q 24 hours
after dialysis.

### Adverse reactions

Abdominal pain or discomfort ▪
aching ▪ arthralgia ▪ arthropathy ▪
burning ▪ chest pain ▪ confusion ▪
constipation ▪ crystalluria ▪

depression ▪ *diarrhea* ▪ dizziness ▪
drowsiness ▪ dyspepsia ▪ edema ▪
eosinophilia ▪ erythema ▪ exfoliative dermatitis ▪ fatigue ▪ flatulence
▪ hallucinations ▪ headache ▪
hypersensitivity reactions ▪
insomnia ▪ interstitial nephritis ▪
joint inflammation ▪ joint or
back pain ▪ joint stiffness ▪ light-
headedness ▪ *nausea* ▪ neck pain ▪
*neutropenia* ▪ oral candidiasis ▪
paresthesia ▪ photosensitivity ▪
pruritus ▪ *pseudomembranous
colitis* ▪ rash ▪ restlessness ▪
*seizures* ▪ *Stevens-Johnson syndrome* ▪ tendon rupture ▪ *thrombocytopenia* ▪ thrombophlebitis ▪
*toxic epidermal necrolysis* ▪
tremors ▪ vomiting

### Nursing considerations

■ Obtain specimen for culture and
sensitivity testing before giving
first dose. Therapy may begin while
awaiting results.

■ Be aware of drug interactions. It
may be necessary to wait up to 6
hours after ciprofloxacin administration before giving another drug
to avoid decreasing drug's effects.
Food doesn't affect drug absorption
but may delay peak drug level.

■ Dilute drug to 1 to 2 mg/ml using
$D_5W$ or normal saline solution.
Infuse over 1 hour.

■ Monitor patient's intake and output and observe for signs and
symptoms of crystalluria.

*(continued)*

■ Long-term therapy may result in overgrowth of organisms resistant to ciprofloxacin.

■ Ciprofloxacin or doxycycline is a first-line therapy for anthrax. Amoxicillin 500 mg P.O. t.i.d. for adults and 80 mg/kg daily in divided doses every 8 hours for children is an option for completion of therapy after clinical improvement.

■ Follow current Centers for Disease Control and Prevention recommendations for anthrax.

■ Pregnant women and immuno-compromised patients should receive the usual doses and regimens for anthrax.

## citalopram hydrobromide
(sih-TAH-loh-pram high-droh-BROH-mighd)

Celexa

Pregnancy risk category: C

### Indications and dosages

**Depression**
■ *Adults:* Initially, 20 mg P.O. once daily, increasing to 40 mg daily after no less than 1 week. Maximum dosage, 40 mg daily.
■ *Elderly patients:* 20 mg P.O. daily with adjustment to 40 mg daily only for patients who don't initially respond to the drug.
*Adjust-a-dose:* For patients with hepatic impairment, 20 mg P.O. daily with adjustment to 40 mg daily only for patients who don't initially respond to the drug.

### Adverse reactions

Abdominal pain • abnormal accommodation • agitation • amenorrhea • amnesia • anorexia • anorgasmia • anxiety • apathy • arthralgia • confusion • coughing • decreased libido • depression • diarrhea • dizziness • dry mouth • dysmenorrhea • dyspepsia • ejaculation disorder • fatigue • fever • flatulence • hypotension • impaired concentration • impotence • increased appetite • increased salivation • *increased sweating* • insomnia • migraine • myalgia • *nausea* • orthostatic hypotension • paresthesia • polyuria • pruritus • rash • rhinitis • sinusitis • *somnolence* • **suicide attempt** • tachycardia • taste perversion • tremor • upper respiratory tract infection • vomiting • weight gain or loss • yawning

### Nursing considerations

■ The possibility of a suicide attempt is inherent in depression and may persist until significant remission occurs. Closely supervise high-risk patients at start of therapy. Reduce risk of overdose by limiting amount of drug available per refill.
■ At least 14 days should elapse between MAO inhibitor therapy and citalopram therapy.
**Watch out!** Don't confuse Celexa with Celebrex or Cerebyx.

# clarithromycin (klah-rith-roh-MIGH-sin)

Biaxin, Biaxin XL

Pregnancy risk category: C

## Indications and dosages

**Pharyngitis or tonsillitis caused by *Streptococcus pyogenes***
■ *Adults:* 250 mg P.O. q 12 hours for 10 days.
■ *Children:* 15 mg/kg/day P.O. divided q 12 hours for 10 days.

**Acute maxillary sinusitis caused by *Streptococcus pneumoniae, Haemophilus influenzae,* or *Moraxella catarrhalis***
■ *Adults:* 500 mg P.O. q 12 hours for 14 days, or two 500-mg extended-release tablets P.O. daily for 14 days.
■ *Children:* 15 mg/kg/day P.O. divided q 12 hours for 10 days.

**Acute worsening of chronic bronchitis caused by *M. catarrhalis,* or *S. pneumoniae;* community-acquired pneumonia caused by *H. influenzae, S. pneumoniae, Mycoplasma pneumoniae,* or *Chlamydia pneumoniae***
■ *Adults:* 250 mg P.O. q 12 hours for 7 days (*H. influenzae*) or 7 to 14 days (others).

**Acute worsening of chronic bronchitis caused by *Haemophilus parainfluenzae* or *H. influenzae***
■ *Adults:* 500 mg P.O. q 12 hours for 7 days (*H. parainfluenzae*) or 7 to 14 days (*H. influenzae*).

**Acute worsening of chronic bronchitis caused by *M. catarrhalis, S. pneumoniae, H. parainfluenzae,* or *H. influenzae***
■ *Adults:* Two 500-mg extended-release tablets daily for 7 days.

**Mild to moderate community-acquired pneumonia caused by *H. influenzae, H. parainfluenzae, M. catarrhalis, S. pneumoniae, C. pneumoniae,* or *M. pneumoniae***
■ *Adults:* Two 500-mg extended-release tablets daily for 7 days.

**Community-acquired pneumonia caused by *S. pneumoniae, C. pneumoniae,* or *M. pneumoniae***
■ *Children:* 15 mg/kg/day P.O. divided q 12 hours for 10 days.

**Uncomplicated skin and skin-structure infections caused by *Staphylococcus aureus* or *S. pyogenes***
■ *Adults:* 250 mg P.O. q 12 hours for 7 to 14 days.
■ *Children:* 15 mg/kg/day P.O. divided q 12 hours for 10 days.

**Acute otitis media caused by *H. influenzae, M. catarrhalis,* or *S. pneumoniae***
■ *Children:* 15 mg/kg/day P.O. divided q 12 hours for 10 days.

**To prevent and treat disseminated infection caused by *Mycobacterium avium complex***
■ *Adults:* 500 mg P.O. b.i.d.
■ *Children:* 7.5 mg/kg P.O. b.i.d., up to 500 mg b.i.d.

## clarithromycin *(continued)*

### *Helicobacter pylori* infection; to reduce risk of duodenal ulcer recurrence

■ *Adults:* 500 mg clarithromycin with 30 mg lansoprazole and 1 g amoxicillin, all given q 12 hours for 10 to 14 days. Or, 500 mg clarithromycin with 20 mg omeprazole and 1 g amoxicillin, all given q 12 hours for 10 days. Or, 500 mg clarithromycin b.i.d., 20 mg rabeprazole b.i.d., and 1 g amoxicillin b.i.d., all for 7 days. Or, two-drug regimen with 500 mg clarithromycin q 8 hours and 40 mg omeprazole once daily for 14 days. Continue omeprazole for 14 additional days.

*Adjust-a-dose:* For patients with creatinine clearance less than 30 ml/minute, cut dose in half or double frequency interval.

### Adverse reactions

Abdominal pain or discomfort ▪ coagulation abnormalities ▪ diarrhea ▪ headache ▪ *leukopenia* ▪ nausea ▪ *pseudomembranous colitis* ▪ rash (pediatric) ▪ taste perversion ▪ vomiting (pediatric)

### Nursing considerations

■ Drug is contraindicated in patients hypersensitive to macrolides and in those also taking pimozide or other drugs that prolong the QT interval or cause arrhythmias.

■ Obtain specimen for culture and sensitivity testing before giving first dose. Therapy may begin pending results.

■ Monitor patient for signs and symptoms of superinfection.

■ Giving clarithromycin with a drug metabolized by CYP3A may increase drug level and prolong therapeutic and adverse effects of the drug given concomitantly.

## clindamycin (klin-duh-MIGH-sin)

clindamycin hydrochloride
**Cleocin HCl, Dalacin C†**
clindamycin palmitate hydrochloride
**Cleocin Pediatric, Dalacin C Flavored Granules†**
clindamycin phosphate
**Cleocin Phosphate, Dalacin C Phosphate Sterile Solution†**

Pregnancy risk category: **B**

### Indications and dosages

**Infections caused by sensitive staphylococci, streptococci, pneumococci, Bacteroides species, Fusobacterium species, Clostridium perfringens, and other sensitive aerobic and anaerobic organisms**
■ *Adults:* 150 to 450 mg P.O. q 6 hours; or 300 to 600 mg I.M. or I.V. q 6, 8, or 12 hours.
■ *Children older than age 1 month:* 8 to 20 mg/kg P.O. daily in divided doses q 6 to 8 hours; or 15 to 40 mg/kg I.M. or I.V. daily in divided doses q 6 or 8 hours.
**Pelvic inflammatory disease**
■ *Adults and adolescents:* 900 mg I.V. q 8 hours, with gentamicin. Continue at least 48 hours after symptoms improve; then switch to oral clindamycin 450 mg q.i.d. for total of 10 to 14 days or doxycycline 100 mg P.O. q 12 hours for total of 10 to 14 days.
**Pneumocystis carinii pneumonia**
■ *Adults:* 600 mg I.V. q 6 hours or 900 mg I.V. q 8 hours, with primaquine.

**CNS toxoplasmosis in AIDS patients, as alternative to sulfonamides with pyrimethamine**
■ *Adults:* 1,200 to 2,400 mg/day in divided doses.

### Adverse reactions

Abdominal pain ● **anaphylaxis** ● diarrhea ● eosinophilia ● jaundice ● maculopapular rash ● *nausea* ● **pseudomembranous colitis** ● **thrombocytopenia** ● thrombophlebitis ● **transient leukopenia** ● urticaria ● vomiting

### Nursing considerations

■ For I.V. infusion, dilute each 300 mg in 50-ml solution, and give no faster than 30 mg/minute (over 10 to 60 minutes). Never give undiluted as a bolus.
■ When giving I.V., check site daily for phlebitis and irritation.
■ Obtain specimen for culture and sensitivity testing before giving first dose. Therapy may begin pending results.
■ For I.M. administration, inject deeply. Rotate sites. Don't exceed 600 mg per injection.
■ I.M. injection may raise CK level in response to muscle irritation.

## clofarabine (kloe-FAR-ah-been)

Clolar

Pregnancy risk category: **D**

### Indications and dosages

**Relapsed or refractory acute lymphoblastic leukemia (ALL) after at least two previous regimens**
■ *Children ages 1 to 21:* 52 mg/m$^2$ by I.V. infusion over 2 hours daily for 5 consecutive days. Repeat about every 2 to 6 weeks as needed. May also give hydrocortisone 100 mg/m$^2$ I.V. on days 1 to 3 of cycle to help prevent capillary leak syndrome.

### Adverse reactions

*Abdominal pain* ● *anorexia* ● *anxiety* ● *arthralgia* ● *back pain* ● **BACTEREMIA** ● **BONE MARROW SUPPRESSION** ● **capillary leak syndrome** ● *constipation* ● *contusion* ● *decreased weight* ● *depression* ● *dermatitis* ● *diarrhea* ● *dizziness* ● *dyspnea* ● *edema* ● *epistaxis* ● *erythema* ● *fatigue* ● **FEBRILE NEUTROPENIA** ● *flushing* ● *gingival bleeding* ● *hand-foot syndrome* ● *headache* ● *hematuria* ● *hepatomegaly* ● *hypertension* ● *hypotension* ● *injection site pain* ● *irritability* ● *jaundice* ● *left ventricular systolic dysfunction* ● *lethargy* ● *limb pain* ● *mucosal irritation* ● *myalgia* ● *nausea* ● **NEUTROPENIA** ● *oral candidiasis* ● *pericardial effusion* ● *petechiae* ● *pleural effusion* ● *pneumonia* ● *pruritus* ● *pyrexia* ● *rigors* ● **RESPIRATORY DISTRESS** ● **SEPSIS** ● *somnolence* ● *sore throat* ● **systemic inflammatory response syndrome (SIRS)** ● *tachycardia* ● *tremor* ● *vomiting*

### Nursing considerations

■ Use very cautiously in patients with hepatic or renal dysfunction.
■ Draw up dose through a 0.2-micron syringe filter and further dilute with $D_5W$ or normal saline solution before infusion.
■ Give over 2 hours with I.V. fluids.
■ Don't give drug with other drugs through the same I.V. line.
■ Monitor patient for dehydration. Give I.V. fluids during the 5-day treatment period.
■ Assess patient for signs and symptoms of tumor lysis syndrome, cytokine release (tachypnea, tachycardia, hypotension, pulmonary edema) that could develop into SIRS, capillary leak syndrome, and organ dysfunction.
■ Stop drug immediately if patient has signs and symptoms of SIRS or capillary leak syndrome.
■ Obtain CBC and platelet counts, and monitor hepatic and renal function regularly during treatment.
■ Stop drug if hypotension develops. If it resolves without treatment, restart clofarabine at a lower dose.

# clonazepam (kloh-NAH-zuh-pam)

Klonopin

Pregnancy risk category: D

## Indications and dosages

**Lennox-Gastaut syndrome, atypical absence seizures, akinetic and myoclonic seizures**
■ *Adults:* Initially, no more than 1.5 mg P.O. daily in three divided doses. May be increased by 0.5 to 1 mg q 3 days until seizures are controlled. If given in unequal doses, give largest dose at bedtime. Maximum dosage, 20 mg daily.
■ *Children up to age 10 or 30 kg (66 lb):* Initially, 0.01 to 0.03 mg/kg P.O. daily (not to exceed 0.05 mg/kg daily) in two or three divided doses. Increase by 0.25 to 0.5 mg q a third day to maximum maintenance dosage of 0.1 to 0.2 mg/kg daily, p.r.n.

**Panic disorder**
■ *Adults:* Initially, 0.25 mg P.O. b.i.d.; increase to target dosage of 1 mg daily after 3 days. Some patients may benefit from dosages up to maximum of 4 mg daily. To achieve 4 mg daily, increase dosage in increments of 0.125 to 0.25 mg b.i.d. q 3 days, as tolerated, until panic disorder is controlled. Taper drug with decrease of 0.125 mg b.i.d. q 3 days until drug is stopped.

**Acute manic episodes of bipolar disorder**
■ *Adults:* 0.75 to 16 mg daily P.O.

**Adjunct treatment for schizophrenia**
■ *Adults:* 0.5 to 2 mg daily P.O.

**Periodic leg movements during sleep**
■ *Adults:* 0.5 to 2 mg P.O. at bedtime

**Parkinsonian (hypokinetic) dysarthria**
■ *Adults:* 0.25 to 0.5 mg daily P.O.

**Multifocal tic disorders**
■ *Adults:* 1.5 to 12 mg daily P.O.

**Neuralgias (deafferentation pain syndromes)**
■ *Adults:* 2 to 4 mg daily P.O.

## Adverse reactions

Abnormal eye movements • agitation • anorexia • ataxia • behavioral disturbances • change in appetite • chest congestion • confusion • constipation • depression • diarrhea • *drowsiness* • dysuria • enuresis • eosinophilia • gastritis • *leukopenia* • nausea • nocturia • nystagmus • palpitations • rash • *respiratory depression* • shortness of breath • slurred speech • sore gums • *thrombocytopenia* • tremor • urine retention • vomiting

## Nursing considerations

■ Drug is contraindicated in patients hypersensitive to benzodiazepines and in those with acute angle-closure glaucoma or significant hepatic disease.

64

## clonazepam *(continued)*

■ Watch for behavioral disturbances, especially in children.
■ Don't stop drug abruptly because this may worsen seizures.
■ Monitor patient for oversedation (especially if elderly).
■ Monitor CBC and liver function test results.

■ Withdrawal symptoms are similar to those of barbiturates.
■ To reduce inconvenience of somnolence when drug is used for panic disorder, giving one dose at bedtime may be desirable.

# clonidine (KLON-uh-deen)

Catapres-TTS
clonidine hydrochloride
Catapres, Dixarit†, Duraclon

Pregnancy risk category: C

## Indications and dosages

**Essential and renal hypertension**
■ *Adults:* Initially, 0.1 mg PO. b.i.d.; then increase by 0.1 to 0.2 mg daily on a weekly basis. Usual range is 0.2 to 0.6 mg daily in divided doses. Or, apply transdermal patch to nonhairy area of intact skin on upper arm or torso once q 7 days, starting with 0.1-mg system and adjusted with another 0.1-mg or larger system.
■ *Children:* 50 to 400 mcg PO. b.i.d.

**Severe cancer pain unresponsive to epidural or spinal opiate analgesia or other more conventional methods of analgesia**
■ *Adults:* Initially, 30 mcg/hour by continuous epidural infusion. Experience with rates greater than 40 mcg/hour is limited.
■ *Children:* Initially, 0.5 mcg/kg/hour by epidural infusion. Dosage should be cautiously adjusted based on response.

**Pheochromocytoma diagnosis**
■ *Adults:* 0.3 mg P.O. as single dose.

**Migraine prophylaxis**
■ *Adults:* 0.025 mg PO, two to four times daily, or up to 0.15 mg PO. daily in divided doses.

**Dysmenorrhea**
■ *Adults:* 0.025 mg PO, b.i.d. for 14 days before and during menses.

**Vasomotor symptoms of menopause**
■ *Adults:* 0.025 to 0.2 mg PO, b.i.d. or 0.1 mg/24-hour patch applied once q 7 days.

**Opiate dependence**
■ *Adults:* Initially, 0.005 or 0.006 mg/kg PO test dose, followed by 0.017 mg/kg PO. daily in three or four divided doses for 10 days. Or, initially, 0.1 mg PO. three or four times daily, with dosage adjusted by 0.1 to 0.2 mg daily. Dosage range is 0.3 to 1.2 mg PO. daily. Stop drug gradually. Follow protocols.

**Alcohol dependence**
■ *Adults:* 0.5 mg PO, b.i.d. to t.i.d.

**Smoking cessation**
■ *Adults:* Initially, 0.1 mg PO. b.i.d., beginning on or shortly before the day of smoking cessation. Increase dosage by 0.1 mg daily, if needed. Or, 0.1 mg/24-hour transdermal patch applied q 7 days beginning on or shortly before the day of smoking cessation. Increase dosage by 0.1 mg/24 hour at weekly intervals, if needed.

## clonidine *(continued)*

### Attention deficit hyperactivity disorder

■ *Children:* Initially, 0.05 mg P.O. at bedtime. May increase dosage cautiously over 2 to 4 weeks. Maintenance dosage, 0.05 to 0.4 mg P.O. daily.

### Adverse reactions

Agitation ▪ anorexia ▪ **bradycardia** ▪ *constipation* ▪ depression ▪ *dermatitis (with transdermal patch)* ▪ *dizziness* ▪ *drowsiness* ▪ *dry mouth* ▪ fatigue ▪ impotence ▪ loss of libido ▪ malaise ▪ nausea ▪ orthostatic hypotension ▪ *pruritus* ▪ rash ▪ *sedation* ▪ **severe rebound hypertension** ▪ urine retention ▪ vomiting ▪ *weakness* ▪ weight gain

### Nursing considerations

■ The injection form concentrate containing 500 mcg/ml must be diluted before use in normal saline injection to yield 100 mcg/ml.

*Alert:* The injection form is for epidural use only; monitor infusion pump and inspect catheter tubing for obstruction or dislodgment.
■ Monitor blood pressure and pulse rate frequently.
■ Elderly patients may be more sensitive than younger ones to hypotensive effects.
■ Noticeable antihypertensive effects of transdermal clonidine may take 2 to 3 days. Oral antihypertensive therapy may have to be continued in the interim.
*Alert:* Remove transdermal patch before defibrillation to prevent arcing.
■ When stopping therapy in patients receiving clonidine and beta-adrenergic blockers, gradually withdraw the beta-adrenergic blocker first to minimize adverse reactions.
■ Don't stop drug before surgery.
**Watch out!** Don't confuse clonidine with quinidine or clomiphene. Don't confuse Catapres with Cetapred or Combipres.

# clopidogrel bisulfate
(kloh-PIH-droh-grel bye-SUL-fayt)

## Plavix

Pregnancy risk category: B

### Indications and dosages

**To reduce thrombotic events in patients with atherosclerosis documented by recent stroke, MI, or peripheral arterial disease**
■ *Adults:* 75 mg P.O. daily.

**To reduce thrombotic events in patients with acute coronary syndrome (unstable angina and non-Q-wave MI), including those receiving drugs and those having percutaneous coronary intervention (with or without stent) or coronary artery bypass graft**
■ *Adults:* Initially, a single 300-mg P.O. loading dose; then 75 mg P.O. once daily. Start and continue aspirin (75 to 325 mg once daily) with clopidogrel.

### Adverse reactions

Abdominal pain ■ arthralgia ■ bronchitis ■ constipation ■ cough-ing ■ depression ■ diarrhea ■ dizziness ■ dyspepsia ■ dyspnea ■ edema ■ epistaxis ■ fatigue ■ flulike syndrome ■ gastritis ■ headache ■ *hemorrhage* ■ hyper-tension ■ pain ■ pruritus ■ purpura ■ *rash* ■ rhinitis ■ ulcers ■ upper respiratory tract infection ■ UTI

### Nursing considerations

■ Drug is contraindicated in patients with pathologic bleeding, such as peptic ulcer disease or intracranial hemorrhage.
■ Platelet aggregation won't return to normal for at least 5 days after drug has been stopped.
■ **Watch out!** Don't confuse Plavix with Paxil.

## co-trimoxazole

sulfamethoxazole and trimethoprim
Apo-Sulfatrim†, Apo-Sulfatrim DS†, Bactrim, Bactrim DS, Bactrim I.V., Cotrim, Cotrim D.S, Cotrim Pediatric, Novo-Trimel†, Novo-Trimel DS†, Nu-Cotrimox†, Roubac†, Septra, Septra DS, Septra I.V., Sulfatrim, Sulfatrim Pediatric

Pregnancy risk category: C

### Indications and dosages

**Shigellosis or UTIs caused by susceptible strains of *Escherichia coli* and *Proteus* (indole positive or negative), *Klebsiella*, or *Enterobacter* species**
■ *Adults:* 160 mg trimethoprim and 800 mg sulfamethoxazole (1 double-strength tablet) P.O. q 12 hours for 5 days in shigellosis and for 10 to 14 days in UTIs. If indicated, give I.V. infusion: 8 to 10 mg/kg/day based on trimethoprim component in two to four divided doses q 6, 8, or 12 hours for 5 days for shigellosis and for up to 14 days for severe UTIs. Maximum dosage, 960 mg trimethoprim (as co-trimoxazole) daily.
■ *Children age 2 months and older:* 8 mg/kg/day based on trimethoprim component P.O. in two divided doses q 12 hours for 5 days for shigellosis and for 10 days for UTIs. If indicated, give I.V. infusion: 8 to 10 mg/kg/day based on trimethoprim component in two to four divided doses q 6, 8, or 12 hours. Don't exceed adult dose.

**Otitis media in patients with penicillin allergy or penicillin-resistant infection**
■ *Children age 2 months and older:* 8 mg/kg/day based on trimethoprim component P.O. in two divided doses q 12 hours for 10 to 14 days.
**Chronic bronchitis, upper respiratory tract infections**
■ *Adults:* 160 mg trimethoprim and 800 mg sulfamethoxazole P.O. q 12 hours for 10 to 14 days.
**Traveler's diarrhea**
■ *Adults:* 160 mg trimethoprim and 800 mg sulfamethoxazole P.O. b.i.d. for 3 to 5 days. Some patients may only need up to 2 days of therapy.
***Pneumocystis carinii* pneumonia**
■ *Adults and children older than age 2 months:* 15 to 20 mg/kg/day based on trimethoprim component I.V. or P.O. in three or four divided doses for 14 to 21 days.
**To prevent *P. carinii* pneumonia**
■ *Adults:* 160 mg trimethoprim and 800 mg sulfamethoxazole P.O. daily; or 80 mg trimethoprim and 400 mg sulfamethoxazole P.O. three times weekly.
■ *Children age 2 months and older:* 150 mg/m² trimethoprim and 750 mg/m² sulfamethoxazole P.O. daily in two divided doses on 3 consecutive days each week.

*(continued)*

*Adjust-a-dose:* For patients with creatinine clearance of 15 to 30 ml/minute, reduce daily dosage by 50%. Don't give to those with creatinine clearance less than 15 ml/minute.

## Adverse reactions

Abdominal pain • *agranulocytosis* • *anaphylaxis* • anorexia • apathy • *aplastic anemia* • arthralgia • aseptic meningitis • ataxia • crystalluria • depression • *diarrhea* • drug fever • *erythema multiforme* • exfoliative dermatitis • fatigue • *generalized skin eruption* • hallucinations • headache • hematuria • hemolytic anemia • *hepatic necrosis* • insomnia • interstitial nephritis • jaundice • *leukopenia* • megaloblastic anemia • muscle weakness • myalgia • *nausea* • nervousness • *pancreatitis* • photosensitivity • pruritus • *pseudomembranous colitis* • pulmonary infiltrates • *seizures* • serum sickness • *Stevens-Johnson syndrome* • stomatitis • *thrombocytopenia* • thrombophlebitis • tinnitus • *toxic epidermal necrolysis* • *toxic nephrosis with oliguria and anuria* • vertigo • *vomiting*

## Nursing considerations

■ Drug is contraindicated in patients hypersensitive to trimethoprim or sulfonamides; in those with creatinine clearance less than 15 ml/minute, porphyria, or megaloblastic anemia from folate deficiency; and in pregnant women at term, breast-feeding women, and infants younger than age 2 months.
■ Obtain specimen for culture and sensitivity testing before first dose. Therapy may begin while awaiting results.
■ Dilute each 5 ml of concentrate for I.V. infusion in 75 to 125 ml of $D_5W$ before administration. Don't mix with other drugs or solutions.
■ Infuse slowly over 60 to 90 minutes.
■ Don't refrigerate; use within 6 hours if diluted in 125 ml and within 2 hours if diluted in 75 ml. Discard solution if cloudiness or crystallization is noted after mixing.
*Alert:* Double-check dosage, which may be written as trimethoprim component.
*Alert:* "DS" product means "double strength."
■ Monitor kidney and liver function test results.
■ Promptly report rash, sore throat, fever, cough, mouth sores, or iris lesions. These early signs and symptoms of erythema multiforme may progress to Stevens-Johnson syndrome, which is sometimes fatal.
■ Watch for signs and symptoms of superinfection.

## cyclobenzaprine hydrochloride
(sigh-kloh-BEN-zah-preen high-droh-KLOR-ighd)

Flexeril

Pregnancy risk category: **B**

### Indications and dosages

**Adjunct to rest and physical therapy to relieve muscle spasm from acute, painful musculoskeletal conditions**

■ *Adults:* 5 mg P.O. t.i.d. Based on response, dose may be increased to 10 mg t.i.d. Don't exceed 60 mg/day. Use for longer than 2 or 3 weeks isn't recommended.
*Adjust-a-dose:* For elderly patients and those with mild hepatic impairment, start with 5 mg and adjust slowly upward. Drug isn't recommended for patients with moderate to severe hepatic impairment.

### Adverse reactions

Abnormal taste ▪ *arrhythmias* ▪ asthenia ▪ ataxia ▪ confusion ▪ constipation ▪ depression ▪ *dizziness* ▪ *drowsiness* ▪ dry mouth ▪ dysarthria ▪ dyspepsia ▪ fatigue ▪ headache ▪ hypotension ▪ insomnia ▪ nausea ▪ nervousness ▪ palpitations ▪ paresthesia ▪ pruritus ▪ rash ▪ *seizures* ▪ syncope ▪ tachycardia ▪ urinary frequency ▪ urine retention ▪ urticaria ▪ vasodilation ▪ vision disturbances

### Nursing considerations

■ Drug is contraindicated in patients with hyperthyroidism, heart block, arrhythmias, conduction disturbances, or heart failure; in those who have received MAO inhibitors within past 14 days; and in those in the acute recovery phase of an MI.
*Alert:* Notify prescriber immediately of signs and symptoms of overdose, including cardiac toxicity.
■ Monitor patient for nausea, headache, and malaise, which may occur if drug is stopped abruptly after long-term use.
**Watch out!** Don't confuse Flexeril with Flaxedil or Floxin.

# dalteparin sodium (dal-TEH-pa-rin SOH-dee-um)

Fragmin

Pregnancy risk category: B

## Indications and dosages

**To prevent deep vein thrombosis (DVT) in patients undergoing abdominal surgery who are at risk for thromboembolic complications**

- *Adults:* 2,500 international units subQ daily, starting 1 to 2 hours before surgery and repeated once daily for 5 to 10 days postoperatively.

**To prevent DVT in patients undergoing hip replacement surgery**

- *Adults:* 2,500 international units subQ within 2 hours before surgery and second dose of 2,500 international units subQ in the evening after surgery (at least 6 hours after first dose). If surgery is performed in the evening, omit second dose on day of surgery. Starting on first postoperative day, give 5,000 international units subQ once daily for 5 to 10 days. *Or,* give 5,000 international units subQ on the evening before surgery, then 5,000 international units subQ once daily starting in the evening of surgery for 5 to 10 days postoperatively.

**To prevent DVT in patients at risk for thromboembolic complications because of severely restricted mobility during acute illness**

- *Adults:* 5,000 international units subQ once daily for 12 to 14 days.

**Unstable angina and non-Q-wave MI**

- *Adults:* 120 international units/kg subQ q 12 hours with aspirin P.O., unless contraindicated. Maximum dosage, 10,000 international units. Treatment usually lasts 5 to 8 days.

## Adverse reactions

*Anaphylaxis* • bleeding complications • ecchymoses • fever • hematoma at injection site • *hemorrhage* • injection site pain • pruritus • rash • *thrombocytopenia*

## Nursing considerations

- **Alert:** If drug is given with epidural or spinal anesthesia or spinal puncture, consider the risk of epidural or spinal hematoma, which may cause long-term or permanent paralysis.
- SubQ injection sites include a U-shaped area around the navel, upper outer side of thigh, and upper outer quadrangle of buttock. Rotate sites daily.
- **Alert:** Drug isn't interchangeable (unit for unit) with unfractionated heparin or other low-molecular-weight heparin.
- Monitor CBC and fecal occult blood tests during therapy.

72

## desirudin (deh-sih-ROO-den)

Iprivask

Pregnancy risk category: C

### Indications and dosages

**To prevent deep vein thrombosis in patients undergoing hip replacement surgery**
■ *Adults:* 15 mg subQ q 12 hours for 9 to 12 days. Give first injection 5 to 15 minutes before surgery, after induction of regional block anesthesia, if used.
*Adjust-a-dose:* If creatinine clearance is 31 to 60 ml/minute, give 5 mg subQ q 12 hours. If clearance is less than 31 ml/minute, give 1.7 mg subQ q 12 hours. Check PTT and creatinine clearance daily. If PTT exceeds two times control, therapy should be stopped until PTT is within two times control; then resume drug at a reduced dose.

### Adverse reactions

*Anaphylaxis* ● anemia ● cerebrovascular disorder ● deep thrombophlebitis ● dizziness ● epistaxis ● fever ● *hematemesis* ● hematuria ● *hemorrhage* ● hypotension ● impaired healing ● injection site mass ● leg edema ● leg pain ● nausea ● *thrombosis* ● vomiting ● wound seeping

### Nursing considerations

■ Reconstitute each 15-mg vial with 0.5 ml of provided diluent (mannitol 3%); then shake vial gently until powder is dissolved. After reconstituted, each 0.5 ml contains 15.75 mg of desirudin.
■ Use reconstituted solutions immediately or store them at room temperature for up to 24 hours protected from light.
■ Use a syringe with a ½" 26G or 27G needle to withdraw all of the reconstituted solution.
■ With the patient lying down, inject entire contents of syringe by deep subQ injection; rotate sites between the right and left thigh or right and left anterolateral and posterolateral abdominal walls.
■ Watch venipuncture sites for bleeding, hematoma, or inflammation.
*Alert:* If drug is given with epidural or spinal anesthesia, be alert for epidural or spinal hematoma, which may cause long-term or permanent paralysis.

# dexamethasone (deks-ah-METH-uh-sohn)

dexamethasone
**Decadron, Dexone, Hexadrol**
dexamethasone acetate
**Cortastat LA, Dalalone D..P, Decaject LA, Dexasone L.A., Dexone LA, Solurex LA**
dexamethasone sodium phosphate
**Cortastat, Dalalone, Decadron Phosphate, Decaject, Dexasone, Hexadrol Phosphate, Solurex**

Pregnancy risk category: C

## Indications and dosages

### Cerebral edema
■ *Adults:* Initially, 10 mg phosphate I.V.; then 4 to 6 mg I.M. q 6 hours until symptoms subside (usually 2 to 4 days); then tapered over 5 to 7 days.

### Inflammatory conditions, allergic reactions, neoplasias
■ *Adults:* 0.75 to 9 mg/day P.O. or 0.5 to 9 mg/day phosphate I.M. Or, 8 to 16 mg acetate I.M. into joint or soft tissue q 1 to 3 weeks. Or, 0.8 to 1.6 mg acetate into lesions q 1 to 3 weeks.

### Shock
■ *Adults:* 20 mg phosphate as single first dose; then 3 mg/kg/24 hours via continuous I.V. infusion. Or, 1 to 6 mg/kg phosphate I.V. as single dose. Or, 40 mg phosphate I.V. q 2 to 6 hours, p.r.n., continued only until patient is stabilized (usually not longer than 72 hours).

### Dexamethasone suppression test for Cushing's syndrome
■ *Adults:* After determining baseline 24-hour urine levels of 17-hydroxycorticosteroids, 0.5 mg P.O. q 6 hours for 48 hours. Repeat 24-hour urine collection to determine 17-hydroxycorticosteroid excretion during second 24 hours of dexamethasone administration. Or, 1 mg P.O. as single dose at 11 p.m. with determination of plasma cortisol at 8 a.m. the next morning.

### Adrenocortical insufficiency
■ *Children:* 0.024 to 0.34 mg/kg or 0.66 to 10 mg/m² P.O. daily, in four divided doses.

## Adverse reactions

Acne • acute adrenal insufficiency (after increased stress or abrupt withdrawal following long-term therapy) • *arrhythmias* • cataracts • cushingoid state • delayed wound healing • edema • *euphoria* • glaucoma • growth suppression in children • headache • *heart failure* • hirsutism • hypercholesterolemia • hyperglycemia • hypertension • hypocalcemia • hypokalemia • increased appetite • increased urine glucose and calcium levels • *insomnia* • menstrual irregularities • muscle weakness • nausea • osteoporosis • *pancreatitis* • paresthesia • peptic ulceration • *pseudotumor cerebri* •

## dexamethasone *(continued)*

psychotic behavior • *seizures* • susceptibility to infections • *thromboembolism* • thrombophlebitis • vertigo • vomiting

### Nursing considerations

■ Drug is contraindicated in patients with systemic fungal infections and in those receiving immunosuppressive doses with live virus vaccines.
*Alert:* After prolonged use, sudden withdrawal may be fatal.

■ For direct injection, inject undiluted over at least 1 minute.

■ For intermittent or continuous infusion, dilute solution according to manufacturer's instructions and give over prescribed duration

■ Give oral dose with food when possible.

■ Give I.M. injection deeply into gluteal muscle. Rotate injection sites to prevent muscle atrophy.

■ Monitor patient's weight, blood pressure, and electrolyte levels.

■ Diabetic patient may need increased insulin; monitor blood glucose levels.

■ Drug may mask or worsen infections, including latent amebiasis.

**Watch out!** Don't confuse dexamethasone with desoximetasone.

# diazepam (digh-AZ-uh-pam)

Apo-Diazepam†, Diastat, Diazemuls†, Diazepam Intensol, Novo-Dipam†, PMS-Diazepam†, Valium, Vivol†

Pregnancy risk category: D

## Indications and dosages

**Anxiety**
- *Adults:* Depending on severity, 2 to 10 mg PO, b.i.d. to q.i.d. or 15 to 30 mg extended-release capsules once daily. Or, 2 to 10 mg I.M. or I.V., q 3 to 4 hours, p.r.n.
- *Children age 6 months and older:* 1 to 2.5 mg PO, t.i.d. or q.i.d.; increase gradually, as needed and tolerated.
- *Elderly patients:* Initially, 2 to 2.5 mg once daily or b.i.d.; increase gradually.

**Acute alcohol withdrawal**
- *Adults:* 10 mg PO, t.i.d. or q.i.d. during first 24 hours; reduce to 5 mg PO, t.i.d. or q.i.d. p.r.n. Or, initially, 10 mg I.M. or I.V.; then 5 to 10 mg I.M. or I.V. q 3 to 4 hours, p.r.n.

**Before endoscopic procedures**
- *Adults:* Adjust I.V. dosage to desired sedative response (up to 20 mg). Or, 5 to 10 mg I.M. 30 minutes before procedure.

**Muscle spasm**
- *Adults:* 2 to 10 mg PO, b.i.d. to q.i.d. Or, 15 to 30 mg extended-release capsules once daily. Or, 5 to 10 mg I.M. or I.V. initially; then 5 to 10 mg I.M. or I.V. q 3 to 4 hours. For tetanus, larger doses, up to 20 mg q 2 to 8 hours, may be needed.

- *Children age 5 and older:* 5 to 10 mg I.M. or I.V. q 3 to 4 hours, p.r.n.
- *Children ages 1 month to 5 years:* 1 to 2 mg I.M. or I.V., slowly; repeat q 3 to 4 hours, p.r.n.

**Cardioversion**
- *Adults:* 5 to 15 mg I.V. within 5 to 10 minutes before procedure.

**Preoperative sedation**
- *Adults:* 10 mg I.M. (preferred) or I.V. before surgery.

**Adjunct treatment for seizure disorders**
- *Adults:* 2 to 10 mg PO, b.i.d. to q.i.d.
- *Children age 6 months and older:* Initially, 1 to 2.5 mg PO, t.i.d. or q.i.d.; increase as needed and tolerated.

**Status epilepticus, severe recurrent seizures**
- *Adults:* Initially, 5 to 10 mg I.V. I.M. Use I.M. route only if I.V. access is unavailable. Repeat q 10 to 15 minutes, p.r.n., up to maximum of 30 mg. Repeat q 2 to 4 hours, if needed.
- *Children age 5 and older:* 1 mg I.V. q 2 to 5 minutes up to maximum of 10 mg. Repeat q 2 to 4 hours, if needed.
- *Children ages 1 month to 5 years:* 0.2 to 0.5 mg I.V. slowly q 2 to 5 minutes up to maximum of 5 mg. Repeat q 2 to 4 hours, if needed.

## diazepam (continued)

**Patients on stable regimens of antiepileptic drugs who need diazepam intermittently to control bouts of increased seizure activity**

■ *Adults and children age 12 and older:* 0.2 mg/kg P.R., rounding up to the nearest available dose form. A second dose may be given 4 to 12 hours later.

■ *Children ages 6 to 11:* 0.3 mg/kg P.R., rounding up to the nearest available dose form. A second dose may be given 4 to 12 hours later.

■ *Children ages 2 to 5:* 0.5 mg/kg P.R., rounding up to the nearest available dose form. A second dose may be given 4 to 12 hours later.

*Adjust-a-dose:* For elderly and debilitated patients, reduce dosage to decrease the likelihood of ataxia and oversedation.

### Adverse reactions

Altered libido • *apnea* • ataxia • blurred vision • *bradycardia* • constipation • *CV collapse* • diarrhea (with rectal form) • diplopia • *drowsiness* • dysarthria • fatigue • hallucinations • headache • hypotension • incontinence • insomnia • jaundice • minor changes in EEG patterns • nausea • *neutropenia* • nystagmus • *pain* • paradoxical anxiety • *phlebitis at injection site* • physical or psychological dependence • rash • *respiratory depression* • slurred speech • transient amnesia • tremor • urine retention

### Nursing considerations

■ Drug is contraindicated in patients with angle-closure glaucoma, shock, coma, or acute alcohol intoxication.

*Alert:* Use of this drug may lead to abuse and addiction. Drug shouldn't be withdrawn abruptly after long-term use; withdrawal symptoms may occur.

*Alert:* When administering I.V., keep emergency resuscitation equipment and oxygen at bedside. Give I.V. dose at no more than 5 mg/minute.

■ Use Diastat rectal gel to treat no more than five episodes per month and no more than one episode every 5 days because tolerance may develop.

■ When using oral concentrate solution, dilute dose just before giving.

■ Monitor periodic hepatic, renal, and hematopoietic function studies in patients receiving repeated or prolonged therapy.

**Watch out!** Don't confuse diazepam with diazoxide.

# digoxin (dih-JOKS-in)

Digitek, Digoxin, Lanoxicaps, Lanoxin

Pregnancy risk category: C

## Indications and dosages

**Heart failure, paroxysmal supraventricular tachycardia, atrial fibrillation and flutter**

*Tablets, elixir*

■ *Adults:* For rapid digitalization, give 0.75 to 1.25 mg PO. over 24 hours in two or more divided doses q 6 to 8 hours. For slow digitalization, give 0.125 to 0.5 mg daily for 7 to 7 days. Maintenance dosage, 0.125 to 0.5 mg daily.

■ *Children age 10 and older:* 10 to 15 mcg/kg PO. over 24 hours in two or more divided doses q 6 to 8 hours. Maintenance dosage, 25% to 35% of total digitalizing dose.

■ *Children ages 5 to 10:* 20 to 35 mcg/kg PO. over 24 hours in two or more divided doses q 6 to 8 hours. Maintenance dosage, 25% to 35% of total digitalizing dose.

■ *Children ages 2 to 5:* 30 to 40 mcg/kg PO. over 24 hours in two or more divided doses q 6 to 8 hours. Maintenance dosage, 25% to 35% of total digitalizing dose.

■ *Infants ages 1 month to 2 years:* 35 to 60 mcg/kg PO. over 24 hours in two or more divided doses q 6 to 8 hours. Maintenance dosage, 25% to 35% of total digitalizing dose.

■ *Neonates:* 25 to 35 mcg/kg PO. over 24 hours in two or more divided doses q 6 to 8 hours. Maintenance dosage, 25% to 35% of total digitalizing dose.

■ *Premature infants:* 20 to 30 mcg/kg PO. over 24 hours in two or more divided doses q 6 to 8 hours. Maintenance dosage, 20% to 30% of total digitalizing dose.

*Capsules*

■ *Adults:* For rapid digitalization, give 0.4 to 0.6 mg PO. initially, followed by 0.1 to 0.3 mg q 6 to 8 hours, p.r.n. and as tolerated, for 24 hours. For slow digitalization, give 0.05 to 0.35 mg daily in two divided doses for 7 to 22 days, p.r.n., until therapeutic levels are reached. Maintenance dosage, 0.05 to 0.35 mg daily in one or two divided doses.

■ *Children:* Digitalizing dose is based on child's age and is given in three or more divided doses over the first 24 hours. First dose is 50% of the total dose; subsequent doses are given q 4 to 8 hours p.r.n. and as tolerated.

■ *Children age 10 and older:* For rapid digitalization, give 8 to 12 mcg/kg PO. over 24 hours, divided as above. Maintenance dosage, 25% to 35% of total digitalizing dose, given daily as a single dose.

## digoxin *(continued)*

■ *Children ages 5 to 10:* For rapid digitalization, give 15 to 30 mcg/kg P.O. over 24 hours, divided as above. Maintenance dosage, 25% to 35% of total digitalizing dose, divided and given in two or three equal doses daily.

■ *Children ages 2 to 5:* For rapid digitalization, give 25 to 35 mcg/kg P.O. over 24 hours, divided as above. Maintenance dosage, 25% to 35% of total digitalizing dose, divided and given in two or three equal doses daily.

*Injection*

■ *Adults:* For rapid digitalization, give 0.4 to 0.6 mg I.V. initially, followed by 0.1 to 0.3 mg I.V. q 4 to 8 hours, p.r.n. and as tolerated, for 24 hours. For slow digitalization, give appropriate daily maintenance dosage for 7 to 22 days p.r.n. until therapeutic levels are reached. Maintenance dosage, 0.125 to 0.5 mg I.V. daily in one to two divided doses.

■ *Children:* Digitalizing dosage is based on child's age and is given in three or more divided doses over the first 24 hours. First dose is 50% of total dose; subsequent doses are given q 4 to 8 hours p.r.n. and as tolerated.

■ *Children age 10 and older:* For rapid digitalization, give 8 to 12 mcg/kg I.V. over 24 hours divided as above. Maintenance dosage, 25% to 35% of total digitalizing dose, given daily as a single dose.

■ *Children ages 5 to 10:* For rapid digitalization, give 15 to 30 mcg/kg I.V. over 24 hours, divided as above. Maintenance dosage, 25% to 35% of total digitalizing dose, divided and given in two or three equal doses daily.

■ *Children ages 2 to 5:* For rapid digitalization, give 25 to 35 mcg/kg I.V. over 24 hours, divided as above. Maintenance dosage, 25% to 35% of total digitalizing dose, divided and given in two or three equal doses daily.

■ *Infants ages 1 month to 2 years:* For rapid digitalization, give 30 to 50 mcg/kg I.V. over 24 hours, divided as above. Maintenance dosage, 25% to 35% of total digitalizing dose, divided and given in two or three equal doses daily.

■ *Neonates:* For rapid digitalization, give 20 to 30 mcg/kg I.V. over 24 hours, divided as above. Maintenance dosage, 25% to 35% of total digitalizing dose, divided and given in two or three equal doses daily.

■ *Premature infants:* For rapid digitalization, give 15 to 25 mcg/kg I.V. over 24 hours, divided as above. Maintenance dosage, 20% to 30% of total digitalizing dose, divided and given in two or three equal doses daily.

*Adjust-a-dose:* Give smaller loading and maintenance doses to patients with impaired renal function.

*(continued)*

# digoxin (continued)

## Adverse reactions

*Agitation* • *anorexia* • *arrhythmias* • blurred vision • diarrhea • diplopia • dizziness • *fatigue* • *generalized muscle weakness* • *hallucinations* • headache • light flashes • malaise • *nausea* • paresthesia • photophobia • stupor • vertigo • vomiting • yellow-green halos around visual images

## Nursing considerations

■ Drug-induced arrhythmias may increase the severity of heart failure and hypotension.

■ When administering I.V., dilute fourfold with D$_5$W, normal saline solution, or sterile water for injection to reduce the chance of precipitation. Infuse drug slowly over at least 5 minutes.

■ Before giving drug, take apical-radial pulse for 1 minute. Record and notify prescriber of significant changes.

■ Excessive slowing of the pulse rate (60 beats/minute or less) may be a sign of digoxin toxicity. Withhold drug and notify prescriber.

■ Monitor potassium level carefully. Take corrective action before hypokalemia occurs.

■ Monitor digoxin level.

**Watch out!** Don't confuse digoxin with doxepin.

# diltiazem hydrochloride
(dil-TIGH-uh-zem high-droh-KLOR-ighd)

Apo-Diltiaz[†], Cardizem, Cardizem CD, Cardizem LA, Cardizem SR, Cartia XT, Dilacor XR, Diltia XT, Tiazac

Pregnancy risk category: C

## Indications and dosages

**To manage Prinzmetal's or variant angina or chronic stable angina pectoris**

■ *Adults:* 30 mg P.O. q.i.d. before meals and bedtime. Increase dose gradually to maximum of 360 mg/day divided into three to four doses, as indicated. Or, give 120 or 180 mg (extended-release) P.O. once daily. Adjust over a 7- to 14-day period p.r.n. and as tolerated up to maximum of 360 mg/day (Cardizem LA), 480 mg/day (Cardizem CD, Cartia XT, Dilacor XR, Dilacor XT), or 540 mg/day (Tiazac).

**Hypertension**

■ *Adults:* 60 to 120 mg P.O. b.i.d. (sustained-release). Adjust up to maximum of 360 mg/day, p.r.n. Or, give 180 to 240 mg (extended-release) P.O. once daily. Adjust dosage, based on patient response, to maximum of 480 mg/day. Or, 120 to 240 mg P.O. (Cardizem LA) once daily. Dosage can be adjusted about every 2 weeks to maximum of 540 mg daily.

**Atrial fibrillation or flutter, paroxysmal supraventricular tachycardia**

■ *Adults:* 0.25 mg/kg I.V. as a bolus injection over 2 minutes. If response isn't adequate after 15 minutes, give 0.35 mg/kg I.V. over 2 minutes. Follow bolus with continuous I.V. infusion at 5 to 15 mg/hour (for up to 24 hours).

## Adverse reactions

Abdominal discomfort ● *acute hepatic injury* ● *arrhythmias* ● asthenia ● *AV block* ● *bradycardia* ● conduction abnormalities ● constipation ● dizziness ● *edema* ● flushing ● *headache* ● **heart failure** ● hypotension ● nausea ● rash ● somnolence

## Nursing considerations

■ Monitor blood pressure and heart rate at start of therapy and during dosage adjustments.
■ Maximum antihypertensive effect may not be seen for 14 days.
■ If systolic blood pressure is below 90 mm Hg or heart rate is below 60 beats/minute, withhold dose and notify prescriber.
**Watch out!** Don't confuse Cardizem SR with Cardene SR.

# diphenhydramine hydrochloride
(digh-fen-HIGH-drah-meen high-droh-KLOR-ighd)

Allerdryl*, AllerMax Caplets, Aller-med, Banophen, Banophen Caplets,
Benadryl, Benadryl Allergy, Compoz, Diphen Cough, Diphenhist, Diphenhist
Captabs, Dormarex 2, Genahist, Hydramine Cough, Nervine Nighttime Sleep-
Aid, Sleep-eze 3, Sominex, Tussstat, Twilite Caplets

Pregnancy risk category: B

## Indications and dosages

**Rhinitis, allergy symptoms,
motion sickness, Parkinson's
disease**

*Adults and children age 12 and
older:* 25 to 50 mg PO, t.i.d. or q.i.d.
Maximum, 300 mg PO. daily. Or,
10 to 50 mg deep I.M. or I.V. Maximum by I.M. or I.V. route, 400 mg
daily.

*Children younger than age 12:*
5 mg/kg/day PO, deep I.M. or I.V. in
divided doses q.i.d. Maximum,
300 mg daily.

### Sedation
*Adults:* 25 to 50 mg PO. or deep
I.M., p.r.n.

### Nighttime sleep aid
*Adults:* 25 to 50 mg PO. at bedtime

### Nonproductive cough (syrup
only)
*Adults and children age 12 and
older:* 25 mg PO, q 4 to 6 hours.
Don't exceed 150 mg daily.

*Children ages 6 to 11:* 12.5 mg
PO, q 4 to 6 hours. Don't exceed
75 mg daily.

*Children ages 2 to 5:* 6.25 mg PO.
q 4 to 6 hours. Don't exceed 25 mg
daily.

## Adverse reactions

*Agranulocytosis · anaphylactic
shock*

*Nausea* · blurred vision
confusion · constipation · diarrhea · diplopia · *dizziness* ·
*drowsiness* · *dry mouth* · dysuria ·
epigastric distress · fatigue ·
headache · hemolytic anemia ·
hypotension · *incoordination* ·
insomnia · nasal congestion ·
nausea · nervousness · palpitations · photosensitivity · rash ·
restlessness · *sedation · seizures*
· *sleepiness · tachycardia ·* thick-
ening of bronchial secretions ·
*thrombocytopenia* · tinnitus ·
tremor · urinary frequency · urine
retention · urticaria · vertigo ·
vomiting

## Nursing considerations

■ Drug is contraindicated in patients
having acute asthma attacks.
■ Alternate injection sites to prevent irritation. Give I.M. injection
deeply into large muscle.
■ Expect to stop drug 4 days
before diagnostic skin testing
because it can prevent, reduce, or
mask positive skin test response.

**Watch out!** Don't confuse
diphenhydramine with dimenhydri-
nate; or Benadryl with benazepril,
Bentyl, or Benylin.

82

## donepezil hydrochloride
(doh-NEH-peh-zil high-droh-KLOR-ighd)

Aricept

Pregnancy risk category: C

### Indications and dosages

**Mild to moderate Alzheimer's dementia**

■ *Adults:* Initially, 5 mg P.O. daily at bedtime. After 4 to 6 weeks, increase to 10 mg daily.

### Adverse reactions

Abnormal crying ▪ abnormal dreams ▪ aggression ▪ anorexia ▪ aphasia ▪ arthritis ▪ ataxia ▪ atrial fibrillation ▪ bloating ▪ blurred vision ▪ bone fracture ▪ bronchitis ▪ cataract ▪ chest pain ▪ dehydration ▪ depression ▪ diaphoresis ▪ *diarrhea* ▪ dizziness ▪ dyspnea ▪ ecchymoses ▪ epigastric pain ▪ eye irritation ▪ fatigue ▪ fecal incontinence ▪ GI bleeding ▪ *headache* ▪ hot flushes ▪ hypertension ▪ hypotension ▪ increased libido ▪ influenza ▪ *insomnia* ▪ irritability ▪ muscle cramps ▪ *nausea* ▪ nervousness ▪ paresthesia ▪ pain ▪ pruritus ▪ restlessness ▪ *seizures* ▪ somnolence ▪ sore throat ▪ syncope ▪ toothache ▪ tremor ▪ urinary frequency ▪ urticaria ▪ vasodilation ▪ vertigo ▪ vomiting ▪ weight loss

### Nursing considerations

■ Monitor patient for evidence of active or occult GI bleeding.
*Alert:* Don't confuse Aricept with Ascriptin.

# dopamine hydrochloride
(DOH-puh-meen high-droh-KLOR-ighd)

Intropin, Revimine†

Pregnancy risk category: C

## Indications and dosages

**To treat shock and correct hemodynamic imbalances, to improve perfusion to vital organs, to increase cardiac output, to correct hypotension**

■ *Adults:* Initially, 1 to 5 mcg/kg/minute by I.V. infusion. Titrate dosage to desired hemodynamic or renal response. Infusion may be increased by 1 to 4 mcg/kg/minute at 10- to 30-minute intervals. Most patients are managed on dosages less than 20 mcg/kg/minute.

## Adverse reactions

**Anaphylactic reactions** ▪ angina ▪ **asthmatic episodes** ▪ azotemia ▪ dyspnea ▪ ectopic beats ▪ headache ▪ hyperglycemia ▪ *hypotension* ▪ nausea ▪ necrosis and tissue sloughing (with extravasation) ▪ palpitations ▪ piloerection ▪ tachycardia ▪ vomiting

## Nursing considerations

■ Drug is contraindicated in patients with uncorrected tachyarrhythmias, pheochromocytoma, or ventricular fibrillation.

■ Dilute with D₅W, normal saline solution, or a combination of D₅W and normal saline solution. Mix just before use.

■ Don't mix other drugs in I.V. container with dopamine. Don't give alkaline drugs, oxidizing drugs, or iron salts through I.V. line containing dopamine.

■ Use a continuous infusion pump to regulate flow rate.

■ Dosages of 0.5 to 2 mcg/kg/minute stimulate dopamine receptors primarily and produce vasodilation of the renal vasculature. Dosages of 2 to 10 mcg/kg/minute stimulate beta receptors for a positive inotropic effect. Higher dosages also stimulate alpha receptors, constricting blood vessels and increasing blood pressure. Most patients are satisfactorily maintained on dosages of less than 20 mcg/kg/minute.

■ Use a central line or large vein, such as the antecubital fossa, to minimize risk of extravasation. Watch infusion site carefully for signs of extravasation; if it occurs, stop infusion immediately and notify prescriber. Extravasation may require infiltrating the area with 5 to 10 mg phentolamine in 10 to 15 ml normal saline solution.

■ Drug isn't a substitute for blood or fluid volume deficit. If deficit exists, replace fluid before giving vasopressors such as dopamine.

## dopamine hydrochloride *(continued)*

■ During infusion, frequently monitor ECG, blood pressure, cardiac output, central venous pressure, pulmonary artery wedge pressure, pulse rate, urine output, infusion site, and color and temperature of limbs.

■ Check urine output often. If urine flow decreases without hypotension, notify prescriber because dosage may need to be reduced.

*Alert:* After drug is stopped, watch closely for a sudden drop in blood pressure. Taper dosage slowly to evaluate stability of blood pressure.

■ Acidosis decreases effectiveness of dopamine.

**Watch out!** Don't confuse dopamine with dobutamine.

# doxazosin mesylate (doks-AY-zoh-sin MES-ih-layt)

Cardura

Pregnancy risk category: C

## Indications and dosages

### Essential hypertension

■ *Adults:* Initially, 1 mg P.O. daily; determine effect on standing and supine blood pressure at 2 to 6 hours and 24 hours after dosing. May increase at 2-week intervals to 2 mg and, thereafter, 4 mg and 8 mg once daily, p.r.n. Maximum dosage, 16 mg daily.

### Benign prostatic hyperplasia

■ *Adults:* Initially, 1 mg P.O. once daily in morning or evening; may increase at 1- or 2-week intervals to 2 mg and, thereafter, 4 mg and 8 mg once daily, p.r.n.

## Adverse reactions

Abnormal vision ▪ *arrhythmias* ▪ arthralgia ▪ *asthenia* ▪ constipation ▪ diarrhea ▪ *dizziness* ▪ drowsiness ▪ dyspnea ▪ edema ▪ *headache* ▪ hypotension ▪ *leukopenia* ▪ myalgia ▪ nausea ▪ *neutropenia* ▪ orthostatic *hypotension* ▪ pain ▪ palpitations ▪ pharyngitis ▪ pruritus ▪ rash ▪ rhinitis ▪ somnolence ▪ tachycardia ▪ vertigo ▪ vomiting

## Nursing considerations

■ Monitor blood pressure closely.
■ If syncope occurs, place patient in recumbent position and treat supportively. A transient hypotensive response isn't considered a contraindication to continued therapy.
**Watch out!** Don't confuse doxazosin with doxapram, doxorubicin, or doxepin. Don't confuse Cardura with Coumadin, K-Dur, Cardene, or Cordarone.

## duloxetine hydrochloride
(doo-LOKS-eh-teen high-droh-KLOR-ighd)

Cymbalta

Pregnancy risk category: C

### Indications and dosages

**Major depressive disorder**

▪ *Adults:* Initially, 20 mg P.O. b.i.d.; then 60 mg P.O. once daily or divided in two equal doses. Maximum, 60 mg daily.

**Neuropathic pain related to diabetic peripheral neuropathy**

▪ *Adults:* 60 mg P.O. once daily.

*Adjust-a-dose:* In renally impaired patients, lower starting dose and gradually increase dosage.

### Adverse reactions

Abnormal orgasm ▪ abnormally increased urinary frequency ▪ anxiety ▪ asthenia ▪ blurred vision ▪ *constipation* ▪ cough ▪ *decreased appetite* ▪ decreased libido ▪ delayed or dysfunctional ejaculation ▪ *diarrhea* ▪ *dizziness* ▪ *dry mouth* ▪ dyspepsia ▪ dysuria ▪ erectile dysfunction ▪ *fatigue* ▪ fever ▪ gastritis ▪ *headache* ▪ hot flushes ▪ hypertension ▪ hypoesthesia ▪ *hypoglycemia* ▪ increased appetite ▪ increased heart rate ▪ increased sweating ▪ initial insomnia ▪ *insomnia* ▪ irritability ▪ lethargy ▪ muscle cramps ▪ myalgia ▪ nasopharyngitis ▪ *nausea* ▪ nervousness ▪ nightmares ▪ night sweats ▪ pharyngolaryngeal pain ▪ pruritus ▪ rash ▪ restlessness ▪ rigors ▪ sleep disorder ▪ *somnolence* ▪ **suicidal thoughts** ▪ tremor ▪ urinary hesitancy ▪ vomiting ▪ weight gain or loss

### Nursing considerations

▪ Drug is contraindicated in patients taking MAO inhibitors and in those with uncontrolled angle-closure glaucoma or creatinine clearance less than 30 ml/minute.

▪ Monitor patient for worsening of depression or suicidal behavior.

▪ Treatment of overdose is symptomatic. Don't induce emesis; gastric lavage or activated charcoal may be used soon after ingestion or if patient is still symptomatic. Contact a poison control center for information.

▪ If intolerable symptoms occur when drug is stopped or dosage is decreased, expect to restart at previous dosage and to decrease even more gradually.

▪ Monitor blood pressure periodically during treatment.

▪ Older patients may be more sensitive to drug's effects than younger adults.

# enalaprilat (eh-NAH-leh-pril-at)

Vasotec

enalapril maleate

Pregnancy risk category: C; D in second and third trimesters

## Indications and dosages

### Hypertension

■ *Adults:* In patients not taking diuretics, initially, 5 mg PO. once daily; then adjusted based on response. Usual dosage range, 10 to 40 mg daily as a single dose or two divided doses. Or, 1.25 mg I.V. infusion over 5 minutes q 6 hours.

*Adjust-a-dose:* If patient is taking diuretics or creatinine clearance is 30 ml/minute or less, initially, 2.5 mg PO. once daily. Or, 0.625 mg I.V. over 5 minutes, and repeat in 1 hour, if needed; then 1.25 mg I.V. q 6 hours.

### To convert from I.V. therapy to oral therapy

■ *Adults:* Initially, 2.5 mg PO. once daily; if patient was receiving 0.625 mg I.V. q 6 hours, then 2.5 mg PO. once daily. Adjust dosage based on response.

### Heart failure

■ *Adults:* Initially, 2.5 mg PO. daily or b.i.d., increased gradually over several weeks. Maintenance dosage, 5 to 20 mg daily in two divided doses. Maximum dosage, 40 mg daily in two divided doses.

*Adjust-a-dose:* If creatinine level is more than 1.6 mg/dl or sodium level is below 130 mEq/L, initially, 2.5 mg PO. daily and adjust slowly.

### Asymptomatic left ventricular dysfunction

■ *Adults:* Initially, 2.5 mg PO. b.i.d. Increase as tolerated to 20 mg PO. daily in divided doses.

## Adverse reactions

Abdominal pain • angina pectoris • **angioedema** • *asthenia* • bone marrow depression • chest pain • decreased renal function (in patients with bilateral renal artery stenosis or heart failure) • diarrhea • dizziness • *dry, persistent, tickling, nonproductive cough* • dyspnea • fatigue • headache • hypotension • nausea • rash • syncope • vertigo • vomiting

## Nursing considerations

■ Closely monitor blood pressure for therapeutic response.

■ **Alert:** Check all labeling carefully. Similar packaging and labeling for enalaprilat injection and pancuronium, a paralyzing drug, could result in a fatal medication error.

■ Monitor CBC before and during therapy.

■ Patients with diabetes, impaired renal function, or heart failure and those receiving drugs that can increase potassium level may develop hyperkalemia. Monitor potassium intake and level.

■ **Watch out!** Don't confuse enalapril with Anafranil or Eldepryl.

88

# enoxaparin sodium
(eh-NOKS-uh-pah-rin SOH-dee-um)

Lovenox

Pregnancy risk category: **B**

## Indications and dosages

**PE and DVT prophylaxis after hip or knee replacement surgery**

■ *Adults:* 30 mg subQ q 12 hours for 7 to 10 days. Give initial dose 12 to 24 hours after surgery, if hemostasis is established. Hip replacement patients may receive 40 mg subQ 12 hours preoperatively. After initial phase of therapy, hip replacement patients should continue with 40 mg subQ daily for 3 weeks.

**PE and DVT prophylaxis after abdominal surgery**

■ *Adults:* 40 mg subQ daily with initial dose 2 hours before surgery. If hemostasis is established, give next dose 24 hours after initial dose and continue once daily, usually for 7 to 10 days.

**PE and DVT prophylaxis in acutely ill patients with decreased mobility**

■ *Adults:* 40 mg subQ once daily for 6 to 11 days.

*Adjust-a-dose:* For patients with creatinine clearance less than 30 ml/minute, give 30 mg subQ once daily.

**To prevent ischemic complications of unstable angina and non-Q-wave MI**

■ *Adults:* 1 mg/kg subQ q 12 hours for a minimum of 2 days, with 100 to 325 mg aspirin P.O. once daily.

**Inpatient treatment of acute DVT with and without PE when given with warfarin**

■ *Adults:* 1 mg/kg subQ q 12 hours; or, 1.5 mg/kg subQ once daily (at same time each day) for 5 to 7 days until INR of 2 to 3 is achieved. Start warfarin therapy within 72 hours of enoxaparin.

**Outpatient treatment of acute DVT without PE when given with warfarin**

■ *Adults:* 1 mg/kg subQ q 12 hours for 5 to 7 days until INR is 2 to 3. Start warfarin within 72 hours of enoxaparin.

*Adjust-a-dose:* If creatinine clearance less than 30 ml/minute, give 1 mg/kg subQ once daily.

## Adverse reactions

**Anaphylaxis** ● **angioedema** ● ecchymoses ● edema ● **hemorrhage** ● injection site irritation ● nausea ● rash ● **thrombocytopenia**

## Nursing considerations

■ Drug is contraindicated in patients hypersensitive to pork products and in those with active bleeding or thrombocytopenia.

# epinephrine (eh-pih-NEF-rin)

epinephrine
**Bronkaid Mistometer*, Primatene Mist**
epinephrine hydrochloride
**Adrenalin Chloride, AsthmaNefrin, EpiPen, EpiPen Jr., microNefrin, Nephron,
Sus-Phrine**

Pregnancy risk category: C

## Indications and dosages

### Bronchospasm, hypersensitivity reactions, anaphylaxis

■ *Adults:* 0.1 to 0.5 ml of 1:1,000 solution subQ or I.M. Repeat q 10 to 15 minutes, p.r.n. Or, 0.1 to 0.25 ml of 1:1,000 solution I.V. slowly over 5 to 10 minutes (1 to 2.5 ml of a 1:10,000 injection). May repeat q 5 to 15 minutes, p.r.n., or follow with a continuous I.V. infusion, 1 mcg/ minute increasing to 4 mcg/minute, p.r.n.

■ *Children:* 0.01 ml/kg (10 mcg) of 1:1,000 solution subQ; repeat q 20 minutes to 4 hours, p.r.n. Maximum single dose, 0.5 mg. Or, 0.005 ml/kg to 0.004 to 0.005 ml/kg of 1:200 Sus-Phrine subQ; repeat q 8 to 12 hours, p.r.n. Maximum single dose, 0.75 mg.

### Acute asthma attacks

■ *Adults and children age 4 and older:* 1 inhalation, repeated once p.r.n. after at least 1 minute; give again for at least 3 hours. Or, 1 to 3 deep inhalations using a hand-bulb nebulizer containing 1% (1:100) solution of epinephrine or 2.25% solution of racepinephrine, repeated q 3 hours, p.r.n

### Cardiac arrest

■ *Adults:* 0.5 to 1 mg I.V., repeated q 3 to 5 minutes p.r.n. Higher-dose epinephrine may be used.

■ *Children:* 0.01 mg/kg (0.1 ml/kg of a 1:10,000 injection) I.V. First endotracheal dose is 0.1 mg/kg (0.1 ml/kg of 1:1,000 injection) diluted in 1 to 2 ml of half-normal or normal saline solution. Subsequent I.V. or intratracheal doses from 0.1 to 0.2 mg/kg (0.1 to 0.2 ml/kg of a 1:1,000 injection) repeated q 3 to 5 minutes p.r.n.

## Adverse reactions

Agitation • altered ECG • anginal pain • disorientation • dizziness • dyspnea • headache • hypertension • nausea • nervousness • palpitations • shock • stroke • tachycardia • tremor • ventricular fibrillation • vomiting

## Nursing considerations

■ Drug is contraindicated in patients with angle-closure glaucoma, organic brain damage, or cardiac dilation and in patients receiving certain general anesthetic agents.

■ 1 mg equals 1 ml of 1:1,000 solution or 10 ml of 1:10,000 solution.

■ **Watch out!** Don't confuse epinephrine with ephedrine or norepinephrine.

# epoetin alfa (ee-POH-eh-tin AL-fah)

**Epogen, Procrit**

Pregnancy risk category: C

## Indications and dosages

**Anemia caused by end-stage renal disease**
■ *Adults:* 50 to 100 units/kg I.V. three times weekly. Nondialysis patients or patients receiving continuous peritoneal dialysis may receive drug by subQ injection or I.V. Maintenance dosage is highly individualized.
*Adjust-a-dose:* Reduce dosage when target hematocrit (HCT) is reached or if HCT rises more than 4 points in 2 weeks. Increase dosage if HCT doesn't rise by 5 to 6 points after 8 weeks of therapy.

**Anemia from chemotherapy**
■ *Adults:* 150 units/kg subQ three times weekly for 8 weeks or until target hemoglobin level is reached. If response isn't satisfactory after 8 weeks, increase dosage up to 300 units/kg subQ three times weekly.
*Adjust-a-dose:* If HCT exceeds 40%, withhold drug until HCT falls to 36%.

**To reduce need for allogenic blood transfusion in anemic patients scheduled to have elective, noncardiac, nonvascular surgery**
■ *Adults:* 300 units/kg subQ daily for 10 days before surgery, on day of surgery, and for 4 days after surgery. Or, 600 units/kg subQ in once-weekly doses (21, 14, and 7 days before surgery), plus one-fourth dose on day of surgery.

**Anemia in children with chronic renal failure on dialysis**
■ *Infants and children ages 1 month to 16 years:* 50 units/kg I.V. or subQ three times weekly. Maintenance dosage is highly individualized.
*Adjust-a-dose:* Reduce dosage when target HCT is reached or if HCT rises more than 4 points in 2 weeks. Increase dosage if HCT does not rise by 5 to 6 points after 8 weeks and is below target range.

## Adverse reactions

Arthralgia ▪ asthenia ▪ clotting of arteriovenous grafts ▪ *diarrhea* ▪ dizziness ▪ *dyspnea* ▪ edema ▪ fatigue ▪ headache ▪ **hyperkalemia** ▪ hypertension ▪ injection site reactions ▪ nausea ▪ pyrexia ▪ rash ▪ **seizures** ▪ vomiting

## Nursing considerations

■ Monitor blood pressure closely.
■ Patient may need additional heparin to prevent clotting during dialysis treatments.
■ Monitor CBC; HCT may rise and cause excessive clotting. Serum creatinine, BUN, uric acid, and potassium levels may also rise.
■ Patients should receive adequate iron supplementation throughout therapy. Patients also may need folic acid and vitamin $B_{12}$.
**Watch out!** Don't confuse Epogen with Neupogen.

# escitalopram oxalate

(ehs-kit-AHL-oh-pram AUKS-ih-layt)

Lexapro

Pregnancy risk category: C

## Indications and dosages

**Treatment and maintenance therapy for patients with major depressive disorder**

▸ *Adults:* Initially, 10 mg P.O. once daily, increasing to 20 mg if necessary after at least 1 week.

*Adjust-a-dose:* For elderly patients and those with hepatic impairment, 10 mg P.O. daily, initially and as maintenance dosage.

## Adverse reactions

Abdominal pain ▪ abnormal dreams ▪ anorgasmia ▪ arthralgia ▪ blurred vision ▪ bronchitis ▪ chest pain ▪ constipation ▪ cough ▪ cramps ▪ decreased libido ▪ diarrhea ▪ dizziness ▪ dry mouth ▪ earache ▪ ejaculation disorder ▪ fatigue ▪ fever ▪ flatulence ▪ flulike symptoms ▪ flushing ▪ gastro-esophageal reflux ▪ heartburn ▪ hypertension ▪ impotence ▪ increased or decreased appetite ▪ increased sweating ▪ impaired concentration ▪ indigestion ▪ insomnia ▪ irritability ▪ lethargy ▪ light-headedness ▪ menstrual cramps ▪ migraine ▪ muscle cramps ▪ myalgia ▪ *nausea* ▪ pain in arms or legs ▪ palpitations ▪ paresthesia ▪ rash ▪ rhinitis ▪ sinusitis ▪ somnolence ▪ *suicidal behavior* ▪ tinnitus ▪ tremor ▪ urinary frequency ▪ UTI ▪ vertigo ▪ vomiting ▪ weight gain or loss ▪ yawning

## Nursing considerations

■ Drug is contraindicated within 14 days of MAO inhibitor therapy.

■ Closely monitor patients at high risk for suicide.

■ Evaluate patient for history of drug abuse and observe for signs and symptoms of misuse or abuse.

■ Periodically reassess patient to determine need for maintenance treatment and appropriate dosing.

# esomeprazole magnesium
(e-soh-MEP-rah-zohl mag-NEE-see-um)

Nexium

Pregnancy risk category: B

## Indications and dosages

**Gastroesophageal reflux disease (GERD), healing erosive esophagitis**

■ *Adults:* 20 or 40 mg P.O. daily for 4 to 8 weeks. Maintenance dosage for healing erosive esophagitis is 20 mg P.O. for no longer than 6 months.

**Symptomatic GERD**

■ *Adults:* 20 mg P.O. daily for 4 weeks. If symptoms are unresolved, may continue treatment for 4 more weeks.

***Helicobacter pylori* eradication**

■ *Adults:* 40 mg esomeprazole P.O. daily, 1,000 mg amoxicillin P.O. b.i.d., and 500 mg clarithromycin P.O. b.i.d., given together for 10 days to reduce duodenal ulcer recurrence.

**To reduce the risk of gastric ulcers in patients on continuous NSAID therapy**

■ *Adults:* 20 or 40 mg P.O. once daily for up to 6 months.

*Adjust-a-dose:* For patients with severe hepatic failure, maximum daily dosage is 20 mg.

## Adverse reactions

Abdominal pain ◦ constipation ◦ diarrhea ◦ dry mouth ◦ flatulence ◦ headache ◦ nausea ◦ vomiting

## Nursing considerations

■ It's unknown if esomeprazole appears in breast milk. Use cautiously in breast-feeding women.

■ Give drug at least 1 hour before meals. If patient has difficulty swallowing the capsule, contents of the capsule can be emptied and mixed with 1 tablespoon of applesauce and swallowed (without chewing the enteric-coated pellets).

■ Patient can use antacids while taking esomeprazole, unless otherwise directed by prescriber.

■ Monitor liver function test results.

# estrogens, conjugated
(ES-troh-jenz, KAHN-jih-gayt-ed)

C.E.S†, Cenestin, Premarin, Premarin Intravenous

Pregnancy risk category: X

## Indications and dosages

**Abnormal uterine bleeding (hormonal imbalance)**
■ *Adults:* 25 mg I.V. or I.M. Repeat dose in 6 to 12 hours, if necessary.

**Vulvar or vaginal atrophy**
■ *Adults:* 0.5 to 2 g cream intra-vaginally once daily in cycles of 3 weeks on, 1 week off.

**Castration and primary ovarian failure**
■ *Adults:* Initially, 1.25 mg Premarin P.O. daily in cycles of 3 weeks on, 1 week off. Adjust dose p.r.n.

**Female hypogonadism**
■ *Adults:* 0.3 to 0.625 mg Premarin P.O. daily, given in cycles of 3 weeks on, 1 week off.

**Moderate to severe vasomotor symptoms of menopause**
■ *Adults:* Initially, 0.3 mg Premarin P.O. daily, or in cycles of 25 days on, 5 days off. Or, 0.45 mg Cenestin P.O. daily. Adjust dosage based on patient response.

**Vulvar and vaginal atrophy caused by menopause**
■ *Adults:* 0.3 mg Cenestin P.O. daily.

**To prevent osteoporosis**
■ *Adults:* 0.3 mg Premarin P.O. daily, or in cycles of 25 days on, 5 days off. Adjust dosage based on bone mineral density.

**Palliative treatment of inoperable prostatic cancer**
■ *Adults:* 1.25 to 2.5 mg Premarin P.O. t.i.d.

**Palliative treatment of breast cancer**
■ *Adults:* 10 mg Premarin P.O. t.i.d. for at least 3 months.

## Adverse reactions

Bloating • *breast tenderness* • depression • *edema* • enlargement of uterine fibromas • flushing • gallbladder disease • *gynecomastia* • headache • **hepatic adenoma** • hirsutism or hair loss • hypertension • impotence • *increased risk of breast cancer, stroke, or endometrial cancer* • menstrual changes • *MI* • nausea • *pancreatitis* • **PE** • *seizures* • testicular atrophy • *thromboembolism* • thrombophlebitis • vaginal candidiasis • vomiting • weight changes • worsening myopia or astigmatism

## Nursing considerations

■ Periodically monitor lipid levels, blood pressure, body weight, and hepatic function.
■ Expect to stop therapy at least 1 month before procedures that prolong immobilization.
■ Glucose tolerance may be impaired. Monitor glucose level closely in patients with diabetes.
**Watch out!** Don't confuse Premarin with Primaxin.

# famotidine (fam-OH-tih-deen)

Mylanta-AR, Pepcid, Pepcid AC, Pepcid RPD

Pregnancy risk category: B

## Indications and dosages

### Short-term treatment for duodenal ulcer
■ *Adults:* For acute therapy, 40 mg P.O. once daily at bedtime, or 20 mg P.O. b.i.d. Healing usually occurs within 4 weeks. For maintenance therapy, 20 mg P.O. once daily at bedtime.

### Short-term treatment for benign gastric ulcer
■ *Adults:* 40 mg P.O. daily at bedtime for 8 weeks.
■ *Children ages 1 to 16:* 0.5 mg/kg P.O. daily at bedtime or divided b.i.d., up to 40 mg daily.

### Pathologic hypersecretory conditions (such as Zollinger-Ellison syndrome)
■ *Adults:* 20 mg P.O. q 6 hours, up to 160 mg q 6 hours.

### Hospitalized patients who can't take oral drug or who have intractable ulcers or hypersecretory conditions
■ *Adults:* 20 mg I.V. q 12 hours.

### Gastroesophageal reflux disease (GERD)
■ *Adults:* 20 mg P.O. b.i.d. for up to 6 weeks. For esophagitis caused by GERD, 20 to 40 mg b.i.d. for up to 12 weeks.
■ *Children ages 1 to 16:* 1 mg/kg/day P.O. in two divided doses, up to 40 mg b.i.d.

### To prevent or treat heartburn
■ *Adults:* 10 mg Pepcid AC P.O. 1 hour before meals to prevent symptoms, or 10 mg Pepcid AC P.O. with water when symptoms occur. Maximum dosage, 20 mg daily. Drug shouldn't be taken daily for longer than 2 weeks.
*Adjust-a-dose:* For patients with creatinine clearance below 50 ml/minute, give half the dose, or increase dosing interval to q 36 to 48 hours.

## Adverse reactions

Acne ▪ anorexia ▪ bone and muscle pain ▪ constipation ▪ diarrhea ▪ dizziness ▪ dry mouth ▪ dry skin ▪ fever ▪ flushing ▪ *headache* ▪ malaise ▪ orbital edema ▪ palpitations ▪ paresthesia ▪ taste perversion ▪ tinnitus ▪ transient irritation at I.V. site ▪ vertigo

## Nursing considerations

▪ Oral suspension must be reconstituted and shaken before use.
▪ Store reconstituted oral suspension below 86° F (30° C). Discard after 30 days.
▪ Assess patient for abdominal pain. Watch for and note blood in emesis, stool, or gastric aspirate.

# fentanyl citrate (FEN-tuh-nihl SIGH-trayt)

Sublimaze

fentanyl transdermal system
Duragesic-25, Duragesic-50, Duragesic-75, Duragesic-100
fentanyl transmucosal
Actiq

Pregnancy risk category: C

## Indications and dosages

**Adjunct to general anesthesia**
*Adults:* For low-dosage therapy, 2 mcg/kg I.V. For moderate-dosage therapy, 2 to 20 mcg/kg I.V.; then 25 to 100 mcg/kg I.V., p.r.n. For high-dosage therapy, 20 to 50 mcg/kg I.V.; then 25 mcg to one-half initial loading dose I.V., p.r.n.

**Adjunct to regional anesthesia**
*Adults:* 50 to 100 mcg I.M. or slowly I.V. over 1 to 2 minutes, p.r.n.

**Postoperative pain, restlessness, tachypnea, and emergence delirium**
*Adults:* 50 to 100 mcg I.M. q 1 to 2 hours, p.r.n.

**Preoperative medication**
*Adults:* 50 to 100 mcg I.M. 30 to 60 minutes before surgery.

**To manage chronic pain**
*Adults:* Apply 1 transdermal system to upper torso. Start with 25-mcg/hour system; adjust dosage p.r.n. System may be worn for 48 to 72 hours. May increase dose 3 days after first dose; then no more often than q 6 days.

**To manage breakthrough cancer pain in patients already tolerating an opioid**
*Adults:* 200 mcg Actiq initially; may give second dose 15 minutes after completion of first dose. Maximum dosage, 2 lozenges per breakthrough episode.

## Adverse reactions

• *Apnea* • *arrhythmias* • *asthenia*
• *clouded sensorium* • *confusion*
• constipation • depression • *diaphoresis* • diarrhea • dizziness
• dry mouth • dyspepsia • dyspnea
• *euphoria* • hallucinations
• headache • hypertension • hypotension • hypoventilation • ileus
• nausea • nervousness • physical dependence • pruritus • *respiratory depression* • *sedation* • *seizures*
• skeletal muscle rigidity (dose-related) • *somnolence* • urine retention • vomiting

## Nursing considerations

**Alert:** High doses can produce muscle rigidity.
■ Monitor circulatory and respiratory status and urinary function carefully.
■ Drug decreases rate and depth of respirations. Monitor arterial oxygen saturation ($SaO_2$). Immediately report respiratory rate below 12 breaths/minute, decreased respiratory volume, or decreased $SaO_2$.
**Watch out!** Don't confuse fentanyl with alfentanil.

## fexofenadine hydrochloride
(feks-oh-FEN-uh-deen high-droh-KLOR-ighd)

Allegra

Pregnancy risk category: C

## Indications and dosages

**Seasonal allergic rhinitis**
- *Adults and children age 12 and older:* 60 mg P.O. b.i.d. or 180 mg P.O. once daily.
- *Children ages 6 to 11:* 30 mg P.O. b.i.d.

**Chronic idiopathic urticaria**
- *Adults and children age 12 and older:* 60 mg P.O. b.i.d.
- *Children ages 6 to 11:* 30 mg P.O. b.i.d.

*Adjust-a-dose:* For patients with impaired renal function or a need for dialysis, give 60 mg daily (adults) or 30 mg daily (children).

## Adverse reactions

Drowsiness • dysmenorrhea • dyspepsia • fatigue • headache • nausea • viral infection

## Nursing considerations

- Expect to stop drug 4 days before patient undergoes diagnostic skin tests because drug can prevent, reduce, or mask positive skin test response.
- No data exist to demonstrate whether drug appears in breast milk; drug should be used cautiously in breast-feeding women. Advise women taking drug to avoid breast-feeding.

# fluconazole (floo-KON-uh-zohl)

Diflucan

Pregnancy risk category: C

## Indications and dosages

### Oropharyngeal candidiasis
- **Adults:** 200 mg PO. or I.V. on first day; then 100 mg once daily for at least 2 weeks.
- **Children:** 6 mg/kg PO. or I.V. on first day; then 3 mg/kg daily for 2 weeks.

### Esophageal candidiasis
- **Adults:** 200 mg PO. or I.V. on first day; then 100 mg once daily for at least 3 weeks and for at least 2 weeks after symptoms resolve.
- **Children:** 6 mg/kg PO. or I.V. on first day; then 3 mg/kg daily for at least 3 weeks and for at least 2 weeks after symptoms resolve.

### Systemic candidiasis
- **Adults:** 400 mg PO. or I.V. on first day; then 200 mg once daily for at least 4 weeks and for 2 weeks after symptoms resolve.
- **Children:** 6 to 12 mg/kg PO. or I.V.

### Vulvovaginal candidiasis
- **Adults:** 150 mg PO. for one dose.

### Cryptococcal meningitis
- **Adults:** 400 mg PO. or I.V. on first day; then 200 mg once daily for 10 to 12 weeks after CSF culture result is negative.
- **Children:** 12 mg/kg PO. or I.V. on first day; then 6 mg/kg/day for 10 to 12 weeks after CSF culture result is negative.

### To suppress relapse of cryptococcal meningitis in patients with AIDS
- **Adults:** 200 mg PO. or I.V. daily.
- **Children:** 3 to 6 mg/kg/day PO. or I.V.

### To prevent candidiasis in bone marrow transplant
- **Adults:** 400 mg PO. or I.V. once daily. Start treatment several days before anticipated agranulocytosis, and continue for 7 days after neutrophil count exceeds 1,000 cells/mm³.

**Adjust-a-dose:** For renally impaired patients, if creatinine clearance is 11 to 50 ml/minute, reduce dosage by 50%. Patients receiving regular hemodialysis treatment should receive usual dose after each dialysis session.

## Adverse reactions

Abdominal pain • *anaphylaxis* • diarrhea • dyspepsia • *headache* • *leukopenia* • nausea • rash • *thrombocytopenia* • vomiting

## Nursing considerations

- Serious hepatotoxicity has occurred in patients with underlying medical conditions; periodically monitor liver function.
- If mild rash develops, monitor patient closely. Stop drug and notify prescriber if lesions progress.
- Risk of adverse reactions may be greater in HIV-infected patients.

98

## flumazenil (floo-MAZ-ih-nil)

Romazicon

Pregnancy risk category: C

### Indications and dosages

**Complete or partial reversal of sedative effects of benzodiazepines after conscious sedation or anesthesia**

■ *Adults:* Initially, 0.2 mg I.V. over 15 seconds. If patient doesn't reach desired level of consciousness (LOC) after 45 seconds, repeat dose. Repeat at 1-minute intervals, if needed, until cumulative dose of 1 mg has been given (first dose plus four more doses). Most patients respond after 0.6 to 1 mg of drug. In case of resedation, repeat dosage after 20 minutes, but never give more than 1 mg at any one time or exceed 3 mg/hour.

■ *Children age 1 year and older:* 0.01 mg/kg I.V. over 15 seconds. If patient doesn't reach desired LOC after 45 seconds, repeat dose. Repeat at 1-minute intervals, if needed, until cumulative dose of 0.05 mg/kg or 1 mg, whichever is lower, has been given.

**Suspected benzodiazepine overdose**

■ *Adults:* Initially, 0.2 mg I.V. over 30 seconds. If patient doesn't reach desired LOC after 30 seconds, give 0.3 mg over 30 seconds. If response is inadequate, give 0.5 mg over 30 seconds. Repeat 0.5-mg doses, p.r.n., at 1-minute intervals until cumulative dose of 3 mg has been given. Most patients with benzodiazepine overdose respond after 1 to 3 mg; rarely, patients who respond partially after 3 mg may need additional doses, up to 5 mg total. If patient doesn't respond in 5 minutes after receiving 5 mg, sedation is unlikely to be caused by benzodiazepines. In case of resedation, repeat dose after 20 minutes but never give more than 1 mg at any one time or exceed 3 mg/hour.

### Adverse reactions

*Abnormal or blurred vision* ■ agitation ■ ***arrhythmias*** ■ cutaneous vasodilation ■ *diaphoresis* ■ *dizziness* ■ dyspnea ■ emotional lability ■ *headache* ■ hyperventilation ■ insomnia ■ *nausea* ■ *pain at injection site* ■ palpitations ■ ***seizures*** ■ tremor ■ *vomiting*

### Nursing considerations

■ Drug is contraindicated in patients hypersensitive to benzodiazepines, patients who show evidence of serious tricyclic antidepressant overdose, and patients who received a benzodiazepine to treat a potentially life-threatening condition, such as status epilepticus or increased intracranial pressure.

■ Monitor patient closely for resedation that may occur after reversal of benzodiazepine effects because flumazenil's duration of action is shorter than all benzodiazepines.

# fluoxetine hydrochloride
(floo-OKS-eh-teen high-droh-KLOR-ighd)

Prozac, Prozac Weekly, Sarafem

Pregnancy risk category: C

## Indications and dosages

**Depression, obsessive-compulsive disorder (OCD)**
■ *Adults:* Initially, 20 mg P.O. in the morning. Maximum dosage, 80 mg daily.
■ *Children ages 8 to 18 (depression):* 10 mg P.O. once daily for 1 week; then increase to 20 mg daily.
■ *Children ages 7 to 17 (OCD):* 10 mg P.O. daily. After 2 weeks, increase to 20 mg daily. Maximum dosage, 60 mg daily.

**Depression in elderly patients**
■ *Adults age 65 and older:* Initially, 20 mg P.O. daily in morning. Doses may be given b.i.d., morning and noon. Maximum, 80 mg daily.

**Maintenance therapy for depression in stabilized patients (not for newly diagnosed depression)**
■ *Adults:* 90 mg Prozac Weekly P.O. once weekly. Start once-weekly dosing 7 days after the last daily dose of Prozac 20 mg.

**Bulimia nervosa**
■ *Adults:* 60 mg P.O. daily in the morning.

**Panic disorder with or without agoraphobia**
■ *Adults:* 10 mg P.O. once daily for 1 week; then increase dosage as needed to 20 mg daily. Maximum dosage, 60 mg daily.

**Premenstrual dysphoric disorder**
■ *Adults:* 20 mg P.O. (Sarafem) daily continuously (every day of the menstrual cycle) or intermittently (daily dose starting 14 days before the onset of menstruation through the first full day of menses). Maximum dosage, 80 mg P.O. daily.
*Adjust-a-dose:* For patients with renal or hepatic impairment and those taking several drugs at the same time, reduce dosage or increase dosing interval.

## Adverse reactions

Anorexia • anxiety • asthenia • constipation • cough • diaphoresis • *diarrhea* • dizziness • drowsiness • dry mouth • dyspepsia • flulike syndrome • *headache* • hot flashes • increased appetite • *insomnia* • muscle pain • *nausea* • *nervousness* • pharyngitis • rash • respiratory distress • sinusitis • sexual dysfunction • *somnolence* • **suicidal behavior** • tremor • upper respiratory tract infection

## Nursing considerations

■ Drug is contraindicated within 14 days of MAO inhibitor therapy.
■ Record mood changes. Watch for suicidal tendencies.
**Watch out!** Don't confuse fluoxetine with fluvastatin or fluvoxamine. Don't confuse Prozac with Prilosec.

# fluticasone propionate
(FLU-tih-ka-sohn pro-PIGH-oh-nayt)

Flonase, Flovent HFA

Pregnancy risk category: C

## Indications and dosages

**Nasal symptoms of seasonal and perennial allergic and nonallergic rhinitis**

*Flonase*

■ *Adults:* Initially, 2 sprays (100 mcg) in each nostril daily or 1 spray b.i.d. Once symptoms are controlled, decrease to 1 spray in each nostril daily. Or, for seasonal allergic rhinitis, 2 sprays in each nostril once daily p.r.n. for symptom control.

■ *Adolescents and children age 4 and older:* Initially, 1 spray (50 mcg) in each nostril daily. If no response, increase to 2 sprays in each nostril daily. When symptoms are controlled, decrease to 1 spray in each nostril daily. Maximum dosage, 2 sprays in each nostril daily.

**As preventative in maintenance of chronic asthma in patients requiring oral corticosteroid**

*Flovent HFA*

■ *Adults and children age 12 and older:* In those previously taking bronchodilators alone, initially, inhaled dose of 88 mcg b.i.d. to maximum of 440 mcg b.i.d.

■ *Patients previously taking inhaled corticosteroids:* Initially, inhaled dose of 88 to 220 mcg b.i.d. to maximum of 440 mcg b.i.d.

■ *Patients previously taking oral corticosteroids:* Initially, inhaled dose of 440 mcg b.i.d. to maximum of 880 mcg b.i.d.

## Adverse reactions

**Angioedema** • bronchitis • **bronchospasm** • cough • cushingoid features • dermatitis • dyspnea • **eosinophilic conditions** • epistaxis • fever • growth retardation in children • *headache* • hyperglycemia • influenza • joint pain • laryngitis • migraine • mouth irritation • muscular soreness • nasal irritation or discharge • nausea • nervousness • *oral candidiasis* • osteoporosis • *pharyngitis* • sinusitis • *upper respiratory tract infection* • urticaria • UTI • viral infections

## Nursing considerations

■ Flovent inhalation aerosol and powder are contraindicated as primary treatment in status asthmaticus.

■ Monitor patient for signs and symptoms of inadequate adrenal response.

*Alert:* Bronchospasm may occur, with an immediate increase in wheezing after dosing. If bronchospasm occurs, treat immediately with a fast-acting inhaled bronchodilator.

# furosemide (fyoo-ROH-seh-mighd)

Apo-Furosemide†, Furoside†, Lasix, Novosemide†, Uritol†

Pregnancy risk category: C

## Indications and dosages

### Acute pulmonary edema
■ *Adults:* 40 mg I.V. injected slowly over 1 to 2 minutes; then 80 mg I.V. in 60 to 90 minutes if needed.

### Edema
■ *Adults:* 20 to 80 mg P.O. daily in the morning, with second dose in 6 to 8 hours; carefully adjusted up to 600 mg daily if needed. Or, 20 to 40 mg I.V. or I.M., increased by 20 mg q 2 hours until desired effect achieved.
■ *Infants and children:* 2 mg/kg P.O. daily, increased by 1 to 2 mg/kg in 6 to 8 hours if needed; carefully adjusted up to 6 mg/kg daily if needed.

### Hypertension
■ *Adults:* 40 mg P.O. b.i.d. Dosage adjusted based on response. May be used as adjunct to other antihypertensives if needed.

## Adverse reactions

Abdominal discomfort ● *agranulocytosis* ● anorexia ● *aplastic anemia* ● azotemia ● blurred or yellowed vision ● constipation ● diarrhea ● dilutional hyponatremia ● dizziness ● fever ● gout ● headache ● hepatic dysfunction ● hyperglycemia ● hyperuricemia (asymptomatic) ● hypocalcemia ● hypochloremic alkalosis ● hypokalemia ● hypomagnesemia ● *leukopenia* ● muscle spasm ● nausea ● oliguria ● orthostatic hypotension ● *pancreatitis* ● paresthesia ● photosensitivity reactions ● purpura ● restlessness ● *thrombocytopenia* ● transient deafness ● vertigo ● vomiting ● weakness

## Nursing considerations

■ Drug is contraindicated in patients with anuria, hepatic coma, or severe electrolyte depletion.
■ To prevent nocturia, give P.O. and I.M. preparations in the morning. Give second dose in early afternoon.
*Alert:* Monitor weight, blood pressure, pulse rate, intake and output, and electrolyte, BUN, and carbon dioxide levels frequently, especially during rapid diuresis.
■ Consult prescriber and dietitian about a high-potassium diet.
■ Monitor glucose level in patients with diabetes.
■ Drug may need to be given I.V. in patients with severe heart failure.
■ Monitor uric acid level, especially in patients with history of gout.
■ Store tablets in light-resistant container to prevent discoloration (doesn't affect potency). Refrigerate oral furosemide solution to ensure drug stability.
**Watch out!** Don't confuse furosemide with torsemide. Don't confuse Lasix with Lonox.

# gabapentin (geh-buh-PEN-tin)

Neurontin

Pregnancy risk category: C

## Indications and dosages

**Adjunctive treatment of partial seizures with or without secondary generalization in adults with epilepsy**

■ *Adults:* Initially, 300 mg P.O. t.i.d. Increase dosage p.r.n. and as tolerated to 1,800 mg daily in divided doses. Dosages up to 3,600 mg daily have been well tolerated.

**Adjunctive treatment to control partial seizures in children**

■ *Starting dosage, children ages 3 to 12:* 10 to 15 mg/kg P.O. daily in three divided doses, adjusting over 3 days until effective.

■ *Effective dosage, children ages 5 to 12:* 25 to 35 mg/kg P.O. daily in three divided doses.

■ *Effective dosage, children ages 3 to 4:* 40 mg/kg P.O. daily in three divided doses.

**Postherpetic neuralgia**

■ *Adults:* 300 mg P.O. once daily on first day, 300 mg b.i.d. on day 2, and 300 mg t.i.d. on day 3. Adjust, p.r.n., for pain to maximum dosage of 1,800 mg daily in three divided doses.

*Adjust-a-dose:* For patients age 12 and older with creatinine clearance of 30 to 59 ml/minute, give 400 to 1,400 mg daily divided into two doses. For clearance of 15 to 29 ml/minute, give 200 to 700 mg daily in single dose. For clearance less than 15 ml/minute, give 100 to 300 mg daily in single dose. Reduce daily dosage in proportion to creatinine clearance (patients with a clearance of 7.5 ml/minute should receive one-half daily dosage of those with clearance of 15 ml/minute). For patients receiving hemodialysis, maintenance dosage is based on estimates of creatinine clearance. Give supplemental dose of 125 to 350 mg after each 4 hours of hemodialysis.

## Adverse reactions

Abnormal thinking ▪ amblyopia ▪ *ataxia* ▪ back pain ▪ constipation ▪ coughing ▪ diplopia ▪ *dizziness* ▪ dry mouth ▪ dyspepsia ▪ *fatigue* ▪ fractures ▪ impotence ▪ incoordination ▪ **leukopenia** ▪ myalgia ▪ nausea ▪ nervousness ▪ nystagmus ▪ peripheral edema ▪ pharyngitis ▪ *somnolence* ▪ tremor ▪ vomiting

## Nursing considerations

*Alert:* Anticonvulsants shouldn't be suddenly withdrawn in patients starting gabapentin therapy.

■ Give first dose at bedtime to minimize drowsiness, dizziness, fatigue, and ataxia.

■ If drug is to be stopped or an alternative drug is substituted, gradually reduce dosage of gabapentin over at least 1 week, to prevent precipitating seizures.

**Watch out!** Don't confuse Neurontin with Noroxin.

# gemfibrozil (jem-FIGH-broh-zil)

Apo-Gemfibrozil, Lopid

Pregnancy risk category: C

## Indications and dosages

Types IV and V hyperlipidemia unresponsive to diet and other drugs; to reduce risk of coronary heart disease in patients with type IIb hyperlipidemia who can't tolerate or who are refractory to treatment with bile-acid sequestrants or niacin

■ *Adults:* 1,200 mg P.O. daily in two divided doses 30 minutes before morning and evening meals.

## Adverse reactions

*Abdominal and epigastric pain* ▪ acute appendicitis ▪ anemia ▪ atrial fibrillation ▪ bile duct obstruction ▪ constipation ▪ dermatitis ▪ diarrhea ▪ *dyspepsia* ▪ eczema ▪ eosinophilia ▪ fatigue ▪ headache ▪ hypokalemia ▪ *leukopenia* ▪ nausea ▪ pruritus ▪ rash ▪ *thrombocytopenia* ▪ vertigo ▪ vomiting

## Nursing considerations

■ Drug is contraindicated in patients with hepatic or severe renal dysfunction or gallbladder disease.
■ Check CBC and liver function test results periodically during the first 12 months of therapy.
■ If no beneficial effects occur after 3 months of therapy, expect prescriber to stop drug.
■ Drug shouldn't be taken with repaglinide or itraconazole.

# gentamicin sulfate (jen-tuh-MIGH-sin SUL-fayt)

Cidomycin†, Garamycin

Pregnancy risk category: D

## Indications and dosages

**Serious infections caused by sensitive strains of *Pseudomonas aeruginosa*, *Escherichia coli*, and *Proteus*, *Klebsiella*, or *Staphylococcus* species**

■ *Adults:* 3 mg/kg I.M. or by I.V. infusion daily in three divided doses q 8 hours. For life-threatening infections, give up to 5 mg/kg I.M. or by I.V. infusion daily in three to four divided doses; reduce dose to 3 mg/kg I.M. or by I.V. infusion daily as soon as patient improves.
■ *Children:* 2 to 2.5 mg/kg I.M. or by I.V. infusion q 8 hours.
■ *Neonates older than 1 week and infants:* 2.5 mg/kg I.M. or by I.V. infusion q 8 hours.
■ *Neonates younger than 1 week and preterm infants:* 2.5 mg/kg I.M. or by I.V. infusion q 12 hours.

**To prevent endocarditis caused by GI or GU procedure or surgery**
■ *Adults:* 1.5 mg/kg I.M. or I.V. 30 minutes before procedure or surgery. Maximum dosage, 80 mg. Give with ampicillin (vancomycin in penicillin-allergic patients).
■ *Children:* 2 mg/kg I.M. or I.V. 30 minutes before procedure or surgery. Maximum dosage, 80 mg. Give with ampicillin (vancomycin in penicillin-allergic patients).
*Adjust-a-dose:* For adults with impaired renal function, doses are determined by gentamicin levels and renal function. To maintain therapeutic blood levels, adults should receive 1 to 1.7 mg/kg I.M. or by I.V. infusion after each dialysis session; children should receive 2 to 2.5 mg/kg I.M. or by I.V. infusion after each dialysis session.

## Adverse reactions

**Agranulocytosis** ▪ **anaphylaxis** ▪ anemia ▪ **apnea** ▪ ataxia ▪ blurred vision ▪ confusion ▪ dizziness ▪ **encephalopathy** ▪ eosinophilia ▪ fever ▪ headache ▪ hypotension ▪ injection site pain ▪ lethargy ▪ **leukopenia** ▪ muscle twitching ▪ myasthenia gravis–like syndrome ▪ nausea ▪ **nephrotoxicity** ▪ numbness ▪ **ototoxicity** ▪ peripheral neuropathy ▪ pruritus ▪ rash ▪ **seizures** ▪ **thrombocytopenia** ▪ tingling ▪ tinnitus ▪ urticaria ▪ vertigo ▪ vomiting

## Nursing considerations

■ Drug is contraindicated in patients with sensitivity to aminoglycosides.
■ Obtain specimen for culture and sensitivity testing before giving first dose. Therapy may begin while awaiting results.
■ Weigh patient and review renal function study results before therapy begins.

*(continued)*

■ Evaluate patient's hearing before and during therapy. Notify prescriber of complaints of tinnitus, vertigo, or hearing loss.

*Alert:* Use preservative-free formulations if intrathecal route is ordered.

■ Obtain blood for peak gentamicin level 1 hour after I.M. injection or 30 minutes after end of I.V. infusion; for trough levels, draw blood just before next dose.

■ Maintain peak levels at 4 to 12 mcg/ml and trough levels at 1 to 2 mcg/ml. The maximum peak level is usually 8 mcg/ml, except in patients with cystic fibrosis, who need increased lung penetration.

■ Monitor urine output, specific gravity, urinalysis, BUN and creatinine levels, and creatinine clearance.

■ Watch for signs and symptoms of superinfection.

## glimepiride (gligh-MEH-peh-righd)

Amaryl

Pregnancy risk category: C

### Indications and dosages

**Adjunct to diet and exercise to lower glucose level in patients with type 2 diabetes mellitus whose hyperglycemia can't be managed by diet and exercise alone**

■ *Adults:* Initially, 1 or 2 mg P.O. once daily with first main meal of day; usual maintenance dosage, 1 to 4 mg P.O. once daily. After reaching 2 mg, increase in increments not exceeding 2 mg q 1 to 2 weeks, based on patient's glucose level. Maximum dosage, 8 mg daily.

**Adjunct to diet and exercise in conjunction with insulin or metformin therapy in patients with type 2 diabetes mellitus whose hyperglycemia can't be managed with the maximum dosage of glimepiride alone**

■ *Adults:* 8 mg P.O. once daily with first main meal of day, used with low-dose insulin or metformin. Increase insulin or metformin dosage weekly, p.r.n., based on glucose level.

*Adjust-a-dose:* For patients with renal or hepatic impairment, initially, 1 mg P.O. once daily with first main meal of day; then adjust dosage p.r.n.

### Adverse reactions

***Agranulocytosis*** ● ***aplastic anemia*** ● asthenia ● changes in accommodation ● cholestatic jaundice ● dilutional hyponatremia ● dizziness ● erythema ● headache ● hemolytic anemia ● ***hypoglycemia*** ● ***leukopenia*** ● morbilliform or maculopapular eruptions ● nausea ● ***pancytopenia*** ● photosensitivity reactions ● pruritus ● ***thrombocytopenia*** ● urticaria

### Nursing considerations

■ Drug is contraindicated in diabetic ketoacidosis and type 1 diabetes mellitus.

■ Glimepiride and insulin may be used together in patients who lose glucose control after first responding to therapy.

■ Monitor fasting glucose level periodically. Also monitor glycosylated hemoglobin level, usually every 3 to 6 months, to assess long-term glycemic control.

■ Use of oral antidiabetics may carry higher risk of CV mortality than use of diet alone or of diet and insulin therapy.

■ **Watch out!** Don't confuse glimepiride with glipizide or glyburide.

## glipizide (GLIGH-peh-zighd)

Glucotrol, Glucotrol XL

Pregnancy risk category: C

### Indications and dosages

**Adjunct to diet to lower glucose level in patients with type 2 diabetes mellitus**

*Immediate-release tablets*

■ *Adults older than age 65:* First dose is 2.5 mg P.O. daily.

■ *Adults age 65 and younger:* Initially, 5 mg P.O. daily 30 minutes before breakfast. Maximum once-daily dosage, 15 mg. Divide doses of more than 15 mg. Maximum dosage, 40 mg daily.

*Extended-release tablets*

■ *Adults:* Initially, 5 mg P.O. daily with breakfast. Increase by 5 mg q 3 months, depending on level of glycemic control. Maximum dosage, 20 mg daily.

*Adjust-a-dose:* For patients with hepatic disease, first dose is 2.5 mg P.O. daily.

### To replace insulin therapy

■ *Adults:* If insulin dosage is more than 20 units daily, start patient at usual dosage in addition to 50% of insulin. If insulin dosage is 20 units or less daily, insulin may be stopped when glipizide starts.

### Adverse reactions

***Agranulocytosis*** ■ **aplastic anemia** ■ cholestatic jaundice ■ constipation ■ diarrhea ■ dizziness ■ drowsiness ■ headache ■ hemolytic anemia ■ *hypoglycemia* ■ **leukopenia** ■ nausea ■ photosensitivity ■ pruritus ■ rash ■ **thrombocytopenia**

### Nursing considerations

■ Drug is contraindicated in patients with diabetic ketoacidosis or type 1 diabetes mellitus.

■ Give immediate-release tablet 30 minutes before meals.

■ Some patients may attain control on a once-daily regimen.

■ Patient may switch from immediate-release to extended-release tablets at the nearest equivalent total daily dose.

■ During periods of stress, patient may need insulin therapy.

■ Patient switching from insulin therapy to an oral antidiabetic should check glucose level before each meal.

**Watch out!** Don't confuse glipizide with glimepiride or glyburide.

## glyburide (GLIGH-byoo-righd)

DiaBeta, Euglucon[†], Glynase PresTab, Micronase

Pregnancy risk category: B

### Indications and dosages

**Adjunct to diet to lower glucose level in patients with type 2 diabetes mellitus**

*Nonmicronized*

■ *Adults:* Initially, 2.5 to 5 mg P.O. once daily with breakfast or first meal. Usual maintenance dosage, 1.25 to 20 mg daily as single dose or divided doses. Maximum dosage, 20 mg P.O. daily.

*Micronized*

■ *Adults:* Initially, 1.5 to 3 mg daily with breakfast or first meal. Usual maintenance dosage, 0.75 to 12 mg daily. Dosages exceeding 6 mg daily may have better response with b.i.d. dosing. Maximum dosage, 12 mg P.O. daily.

*Adjust-a-dose:* For patients who are more sensitive to antidiabetics and for those with adrenal or pituitary insufficiency, start with 1.25 mg daily. When using micronized tablets, patients who are more sensitive to antidiabetics should start with 0.75 mg daily.

**To replace insulin therapy**

■ *Adults:* If insulin dosage is less than 40 units/day, patient may be switched directly to glyburide. If insulin dosage is 40 units/day or more, initially may give 5-mg regular tablets or 3-mg micronized formulation P.O. once daily in addition to 50% of insulin dosage.

### Adverse reactions

***Agranulocytosis*** • **angioedema** • **aplastic anemia** • arthralgia • blurred vision • changes in accommodation • cholestatic jaundice • epigastric fullness • heartburn • hemolytic anemia • ***hepatitis*** • **hypoglycemia** • **leukopenia** • myalgia • nausea • pruritus, rash, or other allergic reactions • ***thrombocytopenia***

### Nursing considerations

■ Drug is contraindicated in patients with diabetic ketoacidosis.

*Alert:* Micronized glyburide (Glynase PresTab) isn't bioequivalent to regular glyburide tablets. Patients who have been taking Micronase or DiaBeta need dosage adjustment.

■ Patients may need insulin therapy during periods of stress.

■ Patients switching from insulin therapy to an oral antidiabetic should check glucose level before each meal.

**Watch out!** Don't confuse glyburide with glimepiride or glipizide.

# heparin sodium (HEH-puh-rin SOH-dee-um)

Hepalean*, Heparin Leo*, Heparin Lock Flush Solution (with Tubex), Heparin Sodium Injection, Hep-Lock

Pregnancy risk category: C

## Indications and dosages

*Note:* Dosage is highly individualized.

**Full-dose continuous I.V. infusion therapy for deep vein thrombisis (DVT), MI, pulmonary embolism (PE)**
- *Adults:* Initially, 5,000 units by I.V. bolus; then 750 to 1,500 units/ hour by I.V. infusion. Titrate hourly rate based on PTT results (4 to 6 hours in the early stages of treatment).
- *Children:* Initially, 50 units/kg I.V.; then 25 units/kg/hour or 20,000 units/m² daily by I.V. infusion. Titrate dosage based on PTT.

**Full-dose subQ therapy for DVT, MI, PE**
- *Adults:* Initially, 5,000 units I.V. bolus and 10,000 to 20,000 units in a concentrated solution subQ; then 8,000 to 10,000 units subQ q 8 hours or 15,000 to 20,000 units subQ in a concentrated solution q 12 hours.

**Full-dose intermittent I.V. therapy for DVT, MI, PE**
- *Adults:* Initially, 10,000 units by I.V. bolus; then titrate according to PTT, and 5,000 to 10,000 units I.V. q 4 to 6 hours.
- *Children:* Initially, 100 units/kg by I.V. bolus; then 50 to 100 units/kg q 4 hours.

**Fixed low-dose therapy for venous thrombosis, PE, atrial fibrillation with embolism, postoperative DVT, and prevention of embolism**
- *Adults:* 5,000 units subQ q 12 hours. For surgical patients, give first dose 1 to 2 hours before procedure; then 5,000 units subQ q 8 to 12 hours for 5 to 7 days or until patient can walk.

**Consumptive coagulopathy (such as DIC)**
- *Adults:* 50 to 100 units/kg by I.V. bolus or continuous I.V. infusion q 4 hours.
- *Children:* 25 to 50 units/kg by I.V. bolus or continuous I.V. infusion q 4 hours. If no improvement within 4 to 8 hours, stop heparin.

**Open-heart surgery**
- *Adults:* For total body perfusion, 150 to 400 units/kg I.V. infusion.

**To maintain patency of I.V. indwelling catheters**
- *Adults:* 10 to 100 units I.V. flush. Use sufficient volume to fill device.

## Adverse reactions

*Anaphylactoid reaction* • cutaneous or subQ necrosis • fever • hematoma • *hemorrhage* • hypersensitivity reactions • irritation • mild pain • *overly prolonged clotting time* • pruritus • rhinitis • *thrombocytopenia* • ulceration • urticaria • *white clot syndrome*

110

## heparin sodium *(continued)*

### Nursing considerations

■ Draw blood to establish baseline coagulation parameters before therapy.

■ Avoid using products containing benzyl alcohol in neonates and pregnant women.

■ Drug requirements are higher in early phases of thrombogenic diseases and febrile states; they are lower when patient's condition stabilizes.

■ Check order and vial carefully; heparin comes in various concentrations.

*Alert:* USP units and international units aren't equivalent for heparin.

*Alert:* Heparin, low-molecular-weight heparins, and danaparoid aren't interchangeable.

■ Inject drug subQ slowly into fat pad. Leave needle in place for 10 seconds after injection; then withdraw needle. Don't massage after injection, and watch for signs of bleeding at injection site. Alternate sites every 12 hours.

■ Measure PTT carefully and regularly. Anticoagulation is present when PTT value is $1\frac{1}{2}$ to 2 times the control value.

■ Monitor platelet count regularly. When new thrombosis accompanies thrombocytopenia (white clot syndrome), expect to stop heparin.

■ Regularly inspect patient for bleeding gums, bruises on arms or legs, petechiae, nosebleeds, melena, tarry stools, hematuria, and hematemesis.

■ Monitor vital signs.

*Alert:* To treat severe heparin overdose, use protamine sulfate. Typically, 1 to 1.5 mg of protamine/100 units of heparin is given if only a few minutes have elapsed; 0.5 to 0.75 mg protamine/100 units heparin, if 30 to 60 minutes have elapsed; and 0.25 to 0.375 mg protamine/100 units heparin, if 2 hours or more have elapsed. Don't give more than 50 mg protamine in a 10-minute period.

# high-molecular-weight hyaluronan
## (HIGH moh-LEK-u-lar high-ah-LOO-roh-nan)

*Orthovisc*

Pregnancy risk category: NR

## Indications and dosages

**To reduce pain caused by osteoarthritis of the knee in patients who haven't responded to nondrug therapy or simple analgesics**

*Adults:* Intra-articular injection (one syringe) into affected knee once weekly for a total of three to four injections.

## Adverse reactions

*Arthralgia* • back pain • bursitis • *headache* • pain at injection site

## Nursing considerations

■ Drug is contraindicated in patients allergic to birds, eggs, feathers, and poultry. Also contraindicated in patients with infection or skin disease in area of injection site or joint.

■ Drug should be given by personnel trained in intra-articular administration.

■ Remove joint effusion before injecting drug.

■ Use an 18G to 21G needle. Using strict aseptic technique, inject contents of one syringe into one knee; if needed, use a second syringe for the second knee.

■ Pain may not be relieved until after the third injection.

■ Don't give less than three injections in a treatment cycle.

■ Inflammation may increase briefly in affected knee in patients with inflammatory osteoarthritis.

■ Don't use drug if original package is open or damaged. Give drug immediately after opening. Store in original package at room temperature (lower than 77° F [25° C]); don't freeze. Discard unused drug.

# hydrochlorothiazide
(high-droh-klor-oh-THIGH-uh-zighd)

Apo-Hydro†, Diuchlor H†, Esidrix, Ezide, HydroDIURIL, Hydro-Par, Microzide, Neo-Codema†, Novo-Hydrazide†, Oretic, Urozide†

Pregnancy risk category: **B**

## Indications and dosages

### Edema
■ *Adults:* 25 to 100 mg P.O. daily or intermittently; up to 200 mg initially for several days until nonedematous weight is attained.

### Hypertension
■ *Adults:* 12.5 to 50 mg P.O. once daily. Increase or decrease daily dosage based on blood pressure.
■ *Children ages 2 to 12:* 2.2 mg/kg P.O. or 60 mg/m$^2$ P.O. daily in two divided doses. Usual dosage range, 37.5 to 100 mg daily.
■ *Children ages 6 months to 2 years:* 2.2 mg/kg P.O. or 60 mg/m$^2$ P.O. daily in two divided doses. Usual dosage range, 12.5 to 37.5 mg daily.
■ *Children younger than age 6 months:* Up to 3.3 mg/kg P.O. daily in two divided doses.

## Adverse reactions

Abdominal pain • *agranulocytosis* • allergic myocarditis • alopecia • *anaphylactic reaction* • anorexia • *aplastic anemia* • constipation • dermatitis • diarrhea • dizziness • epigastric distress • gout • headache • hemolytic anemia • hyperglycemia • hypersensitivity reactions • hypokalemia • hyperuricemia (asymptomatic) • interstitial nephritis • jaundice • *leukopenia* • muscle cramps • nausea • orthostatic hypotension • *pancreatitis* • paresthesia • photosensitivity reactions • pneumonitis • purpura • rash • *renal failure* • restlessness • *respiratory distress* • *thrombocytopenia* • vasculitis • vertigo • vomiting • weakness

## Nursing considerations

■ Drug is contraindicated in patients with anuria, hepatic coma, or hypersensitivity to other thiazides or sulfonamide derivatives.
■ To prevent nocturia, give drug in the morning.
■ Monitor fluid intake and output, weight, blood pressure, and BUN, creatinine, and electrolyte levels.
■ To prevent potassium loss, drug may be used with a potassium-sparing diuretic.
■ Consult prescriber and dietitian about a high-potassium diet.
■ Monitor uric acid level, especially in patients with history of gout.
■ Monitor glucose level, especially in patients with diabetes.
■ Monitor elderly patients, who are especially susceptible to excessive diuresis.
■ In patients with hypertension, therapeutic response may be delayed several weeks.

# hydrocortisone (high-droh-KOR-tuh-sohn)

Cortef, Cortenema, Hydrocortone
Anusol-HC, Anusol-HC, Cortifoam, Proctocort
*hydrocortisone acetate*
Cortef
*hydrocortisone cypionate*
*hydrocortisone sodium phosphate*
*hydrocortisone sodium succinate*
A-Hydrocort, Solu-Cortef

Pregnancy risk category: C

## Indications and dosages

**Severe inflammation, adrenal insufficiency**
■ *Adults:* 5 to 30 mg PO. b.i.d. t.i.d., or q.i.d. (up to 80 mg q.i.d. in acute situations) Or, initially, 100 to 500 mg succinate I.M. or I.V.; then 50 to 100 mg I.M., as indicated. Or, 15 to 240 mg phosphate I.M., subQ, or I.V. daily in divided doses q 12 hours. Or, 5 to 75 mg acetate into joints or soft tissue, repeated at 3 to 5 days for bursae and 1 to 4 weeks for joints. Dosage varies with size of joint.

**Shock**
■ *Adults:* Initially, 50 mg/kg succinate I.V., repeated in 4 hours; repeat dosage q 24 hours, p.r.n. Or, 100 to 500 mg to 2 g q 2 to 6 hours, continued until patient is stabilized (usually not longer than 48 to 72 hours).
■ *Children:* 0.16 to 1 mg/kg or 6 to 30 mg/m² I.M. (phosphate or succinate) or I.V. (succinate) once or twice daily.

**Adjunct treatment for ulcerative colitis and proctitis**
■ *Adults:* 1 enema (100 mg) PR. nightly for 21 days. Or, 1 applicatorful (90-mg foam) PR. daily or b.i.d. for 14 to 21 days. Or, 25 mg rectal suppository b.i.d. for 2 weeks. For severe proctitis, 25 mg PR. t.i.d. or 50 mg PR. b.i.d.

## Adverse reactions

Acne • **adrenal insufficiency with increased stress or following abrupt withdrawal after long-term therapy** • **arrhythmias** • carbohydrate intolerance • cataracts • cushingoid state • delayed wound healing • easy bruising • edema • **euphoria** • GI irritation • glaucoma • growth suppression in children • headache • **heart failure** • hirsutism • hypercholesterolemia • hyperglycemia • hypertension • hypocalcemia • hypokalemia • increased appetite • increased urine calcium level • **insomnia** • menstrual irregularities • muscle weakness • nausea • osteoporosis • **pancreatitis** • paresthesia • peptic ulceration • **pseudotumor cerebri** • psychotic behavior • **seizures**

## hydrocortisone (continued)

• skin eruptions • susceptibility to infections • **thromboembolism** • thrombophlebitis • vertigo • vomiting

#### After abrupt withdrawal

Anorexia • arthralgia • **death** • depression • dizziness • dyspnea • fainting • fatigue • fever • **hypoglycemia** • lethargy • orthostatic hypotension • rebound inflammation • weakness

### Nursing considerations

■ Drug is contraindicated in patients with systemic fungal infections and in premature infants (hydrocortisone sodium succinate).
■ Determine whether patient is sensitive to other corticosteroids.
■ For better results and less toxicity, give a once-daily dose in the morning.
■ Give oral dose with food when possible. Patient may need medication to prevent GI irritation.
*Alert:* Salt formulations aren't interchangeable.
■ Give I.M. injection deeply into gluteal muscle. Rotate injection sites to prevent muscle atrophy. Avoid subQ injection because atrophy and sterile abscesses may occur.
■ Injectable forms aren't used for alternate-day therapy.

*Alert:* Only hydrocortisone sodium phosphate and sodium succinate can be given I.V.
■ Enema may produce systemic effects. If enema therapy must exceed 21 days, expect to stop therapy gradually.
■ High-dose therapy usually isn't continued beyond 48 hours.
■ Monitor patient's weight, blood pressure, and electrolyte levels.
■ Unless contraindicated, give a low-sodium diet that's high in potassium and protein. Give potassium supplements.
■ Drug may mask or worsen infections, including latent amebiasis.
■ Stress (fever, trauma, surgery, and emotional problems) may increase adrenal insufficiency. Expect to increase dosage if patient is experiencing stress.
■ Watch for depression or psychotic episodes, especially during high-dose therapy.
■ Patients with diabetes may need increased insulin; monitor glucose level.
■ Periodic measurement of growth and development may be needed during high-dose or prolonged therapy in children.
**Watch out!** Don't confuse hydrocortisone with hydroxychloroquine. Don't confuse Solu-Cortef with Solu-Medrol.

# hydromorphone hydrochloride
(high-droh-MOR-fohn high-droh-KLOR-ighd)

Dilaudid, Dilaudid-5, Dilaudid-HP

Pregnancy risk category: C

## Indications and dosages

### Moderate to severe pain
■ *Adults:* 2 to 4 mg PO. q 4 to 6 hours, p.r.n. For more severe pain, may use doses higher than 4 mg q 4 to 6 hours, p.r.n. Or, 2 to 4 mg I.M., subQ, or I.V. (slowly over at least 2 to 5 minutes) q 4 to 6 hours, p.r.n. Or, 3 mg suppository PR. q 6 to 8 hours, p.r.n. (Give 1 to 14 mg Dilaudid-HP subQ or I.M. q 4 to 6 hours.)

### Cough
■ *Adults and children older than age 12:* 1 mg cough syrup PO. q 3 to 4 hours, p.r.n.
■ *Children ages 6 to 12:* 0.5 mg cough syrup PO. q 3 to 4 hours, p.r.n.

## Nursing considerations
■ Drug is contraindicated in patients with intracranial lesions caused by increased intracranial pressure and whenever ventilator function is depressed, such as in status asthmaticus, COPD, cor pulmonale, and kyphoscoliosis.
■ *Alert:* Cough syrup may contain tartrazine.
■ Reassess patient's level of pain at least 15 and 30 minutes after administration.
■ Monitor respiratory and circulatory status and bowel function; keep opioid antagonist (naloxone) available.

**Watch out!** Don't confuse hydromorphone with morphine or oxymorphone. Don't confuse Dilaudid with Dilantin.

## Adverse reactions
Blurred vision ∙ *bradycardia* ∙ *bronchospasm* ∙ clouded sensorium ∙ constipation ∙ diaphoresis ∙ diplopia ∙ dizziness ∙ dry mouth ∙ euphoria ∙ flushing ∙ ileus ∙ hypotension ∙ induration ∙ nausea ∙ nystagmus ∙ physical dependence ∙ pruritus ∙ *respiratory depression* ∙ sedation ∙ somnolence ∙ urine retention ∙ vomiting

# hydroxyzine (high-DROKS-ih-zeen)

hydroxyzine hydrochloride
**Anx, Apo-Hydroxyzine†, Atarax, Novo-Hydroxyzin†, PMS-Hydroxyzine†, Vistaril**
hydroxyzine pamoate
**Vistaril**

Pregnancy risk category: X

## Indications and dosages

**Anxiety**
- *Adults:* 50 to 100 mg P.O. q.i.d.
- *Children age 6 and older:* 50 to 100 mg P.O. daily in divided doses.
- *Children younger than age 6:* 50 mg P.O. daily in divided doses.

**Preoperative and postoperative adjunctive therapy for sedation**
- *Adults:* 25 to 100 mg I.M. or 50 to 100 mg P.O.
- *Children:* 1.1 mg/kg I.M. or 0.6 mg/kg P.O.

**Pruritus from allergies**
- *Adults:* 25 mg P.O. t.i.d. or q.i.d.
- *Children age 6 and older:* 50 to 100 mg P.O. daily in divided doses.
- *Children younger than age 6:* 50 mg P.O. daily in divided doses.

**Psychiatric and emotional emergencies, including acute alcoholism**
- *Adults:* 50 to 100 mg I.M. q 4 to 6 hours, p.r.n.

**Nausea and vomiting (excluding nausea and vomiting of pregnancy)**
- *Adults:* 25 to 100 mg I.M.
- *Children:* 1.1 mg/kg I.M.

**Antepartum and postpartum adjunctive therapy**
- *Adults:* 25 to 100 mg I.M.

## Adverse reactions

Constipation • *dry mouth* • *drowsiness* • hypersensitivity reactions • involuntary motor activity • pain at I.M. injection site

## Nursing considerations

- Parenteral form is for I.M. use only, preferably by Z-track injection. Never give drug I.V. or subQ.
- Aspirate I.M. injection carefully to prevent inadvertent intravascular injection. Inject deeply into a large muscle.
- If patient is taking other CNS drugs, observe for oversedation.
  **Watch out!** Don't confuse hydroxyzine with hydralazine or hydroxyurea.

## ibuprofen (igh-byoo-PROH-fen)

Advil, Apo-Ibuprofen†, Bayer Select Ibuprofen Pain Relief Formula, Children's Advil, Children's Motrin, Excedrin IB, Genpril, Haltran, Ibutab, Medipren, Menadol, Midol IB, Motrin, Novo-Profen†, Nuprin, Pamprin-IB, Rufen, Saleto, Trendar

Pregnancy risk category: **B; D** in third trimester

### Indications and dosages

**Rheumatoid arthritis, arthritis, osteoarthritis**
▪ *Adults:* 300 to 800 mg P.O. t.i.d. or q.i.d. Maximum dosage, 3.2 g daily.

**Mild to moderate pain, dysmenorrhea**
▪ *Adults:* 400 mg P.O. q 4 to 6 hours, p.r.n.

**Fever**
▪ *Adults:* 200 to 400 mg P.O. q 4 to 6 hours, for no longer than 3 days. Maximum dosage, 1.2 g daily.
▪ *Children ages 6 months to 12 years:* If child's temperature is below 102.5° F (39.2° C), give 5 mg/kg P.O. q 6 to 8 hours. Treat higher temperatures with 10 mg/kg q 6 to 8 hours. Maximum dosage, 40 mg/kg daily.

**Juvenile arthritis**
▪ *Children:* 30 to 40 mg/kg P.O. daily in three or four divided doses. Maximum dosage, 50 mg/kg daily.

### Adverse reactions

Abdominal pain ▪ *acute renal failure* ▪ *agranulocytosis* ▪ anemia ▪ *aplastic anemia* ▪ *aseptic meningitis* ▪ azotemia ▪ bloating ▪ *bronchospasm* ▪ constipation ▪ cystitis ▪ decreased appetite ▪ diarrhea ▪ dizziness ▪ dyspepsia ▪ edema ▪ epigastric distress ▪ flatulence ▪ fluid retention ▪ headache ▪ heartburn ▪ hematuria ▪ *hyperkalemia* ▪ *hypoglycemia* ▪ *leukopenia* ▪ nausea ▪ nervousness ▪ *neutropenia* ▪ occult blood loss ▪ *pancytopenia* ▪ peptic ulceration ▪ peripheral edema ▪ prolonged bleeding time ▪ pruritus ▪ rash ▪ *Stevens-Johnson syndrome* ▪ *thrombocytopenia* ▪ tinnitus ▪ urticaria

### Nursing considerations

▪ Drug is contraindicated in patients with nasal polyps, angioedema, or bronchospastic reaction to aspirin or other NSAIDs.
▪ Check renal and hepatic function periodically in patients on long-term therapy.
▪ NSAIDs may mask signs and symptoms of infection.
▪ Serious GI toxicity can occur in patient taking NSAIDs, despite lack of symptoms.
▪ It may take 1 or 2 weeks before full anti-inflammatory effects are evident.
▪ If patient consumes three or more alcoholic drinks per day, use of ibuprofen may lead to stomach bleeding.
**Watch out!** Don't confuse Trendar with Trandate.

## infliximab (in-FLIX-i-mab)

Remicade

Pregnancy risk category: B

### Indications and dosages

**Moderately to severely active Crohn's disease; reduction in the number of draining enterocutaneous and rectovaginal fistulas and maintenance of fistula closure in patients with fistulizing Crohn's disease**

■ *Adults:* 5 mg/kg I.V. infused over not less than 2 hours, given as an induction regimen at 0, 2, and 6 weeks, followed by 5 mg/kg every 8 thereafter. For patients who respond and then lose their response, consider 10 mg/kg. If no response by week 14, patient is unlikely to respond.

**Moderately to severely active rheumatoid arthritis (with methotrexate)**

■ *Adults:* 3 mg/kg I.V. infused over at least 2 hours. Give additional doses of 3 mg/kg at 2 and 6 weeks after first infusion and every 8 weeks thereafter. May increase dosage up to 10 mg/kg, or doses may be given every 4 weeks if response is inadequate.

### Adverse reactions

Abscess ▪ *abdominal pain* ▪ acne ▪ alopecia ▪ anemia ▪ *arthralgia* ▪ arthritis ▪ *back pain* ▪ bronchitis ▪ candidiasis ▪ chest pain ▪ chills ▪ conjunctivitis ▪ constipation ▪ *cough* ▪ depression ▪ diaphoresis ▪ *diarrhea* ▪ dizziness ▪ dry skin ▪ *dyspepsia* ▪ dyspnea ▪ dysuria ▪ ecchymosis ▪ eczema ▪ erythema ▪ erythematous rash ▪ *fatigue* ▪ fever ▪ flatulence ▪ flulike syndrome ▪ flushing ▪ *headache* ▪ hematoma ▪ hot flashes ▪ *hypertension* ▪ hypotension ▪ increased urinary frequency ▪ insomnia ▪ ***intestinal obstruction*** ▪ **leukopenia** ▪ maculopapular rash ▪ malaise ▪ myalgia ▪ *nausea* ▪ **neutropenia** ▪ pain ▪ **pancytopenia** ▪ papular rash ▪ pericardial effusion ▪ peripheral edema ▪ *pharyngitis* ▪ pruritus ▪ *rash* ▪ respiratory tract allergic reaction ▪ *rhinitis* ▪ *sinusitis* ▪ systemic and cutaneous vasculitis ▪ tachycardia ▪ ***thrombocytopenia*** ▪ toothache ▪ ulcerative stomatitis ▪ *upper respiratory tract infection* ▪ urticaria ▪ *UTI* ▪ vomiting

### Nursing considerations

*Alert:* Watch for signs of infusion-related reaction, including fever, chills, dyspnea, and chest pain, during administration and for 2 hours afterward. If an infusion-related reaction occurs, stop drug and notify prescriber.

■ Monitor patient for autoimmune antibodies, lupus-like syndrome, lymphoma, and infection.

■ Evaluate patient for latent tuberculosis infection prior to starting therapy.

# insulin glulisine (rDNA origin) injection
(IN-suh-lin GLOO-lih-seen)

Apidra

Pregnancy risk category: C

## Indications and dosages

### Diabetes mellitus
■ *Adults:* Individualize dosage. Give by subQ injection within 15 minutes before a meal. If regimen also includes a longer-acting insulin or basal insulin analogue, give within 20 minutes after meal starts. Or, give drug as continuous subQ infusion using an external infusion pump.

## Adverse reactions

Allergic reaction ● **anaphylaxis** ● **hypoglycemia** ● *injection site reaction* ● insulin antibody production ● lipodystrophy ● pruritus ● rash

## Nursing considerations

■ Use with a longer-acting or basal insulin analogue.
*Alert:* Insulin glulisine has a more rapid onset and shorter duration of action than regular human insulin. Give within 15 minutes before or immediately after a meal.
■ Don't mix insulin glulisine in a syringe with other insulins except NPH.
■ When used in an external subQ infusion pump, don't mix insulin glulisine with other insulins or with a diluent.
■ Changes in insulin strength, manufacturer, type, or species and changes in patient's physical activity or usual meal plan may require a dosage adjustment.
■ Insulin requirements may be altered during illness, emotional disturbances, or stress.
■ Monitor patient for lipodystrophy at injection site; it may delay insulin absorption.

## insulins (IN-suh-linz)

insulin (regular)
**Humulin R, Humulin R Regular U-500 (concentrated), Iletin II Regular, Novolin R, Novolin R PenFill, Novolin R Prefilled, Velosulin BR**
insulin (lispro)
**Humalog**
insulin lispro protamine and insulin lispro
**Humalog Mix 75/25**
insulin zinc suspension
**Humulin L, Lente Iletin II**
extended zinc insulin suspension
**Humulin U Ultralente**
isophane insulin suspension
**Humulin N, Novolin N, Novolin N PenFill, Novolin N Prefilled, NPH Iletin II**
isophane insulin suspension and insulin injection
**Humulin 70/30, Novolin 70/30, Novolin 70/30 PenFill, Novolin 70/30 Prefilled, Humulin 50/50**

Pregnancy risk category: **B**

### Indications and dosages

**Moderate to severe diabetic ketoacidosis (DKA) or hyperosmolar hyperglycemia (regular insulin)**
■ *Adults older than age 20:* Give loading dose of 0.15 unit/kg I.V. direct injection, followed by 0.1 unit/kg/hour as a continuous infusion. Decrease infusion rate to 0.05 to 0.1 unit/kg/hour when glucose level reaches 250 to 300 mg/dl. Start infusion of $D_5W$ in half-normal saline solution separately from insulin infusion when glucose level is 150 to 200 mg/dl in patients with DKA or 250 to 300 mg/dl in those with hyperosmolar hyperglycemia. Give dose of insulin subQ 1 to 2 hours before stopping insulin infusion. (Intermediate-acting insulin is recommended.)

■ *Adults and children age 20 and younger:* Loading dose isn't recommended. Begin therapy at 0.1 unit/kg/hour by I.V. infusion. When the patient's condition improves, decrease insulin infusion rate to 0.05 unit/kg/hour. Start infusion of $D_5W$ in half-normal saline solution separately from insulin infusion when glucose level is 250 mg/dl.
**Mild DKA (regular insulin)**
■ *Adults older than age 20:* Give loading dose of 0.4 to 0.6 unit/kg divided in two equal parts, with half the dose given by direct I.V. injection and half given I.M. or subQ. Subsequent doses can be based on 0.1 unit/kg/hour I.M. or subQ.
**Newly diagnosed diabetes mellitus (regular insulin)**
■ *Adults older than age 20:* Individualize dosage. Initially, 0.5 to 1 unit/kg/day subQ as part of a regimen
*(continued)*

with short-acting and long-acting insulin therapy.

■ *Adults and children age 20 and younger:* Individualize dosage. Initially, 0.1 to 0.25 unit/kg subQ q 6 to 8 hours for 24 hours; then adjust accordingly.

**Control of hyperglycemia in patients with type 1 diabetes mellitus (Humalog and longer-acting insulin)**

■ *Adults:* Dosage varies and must be determined by prescriber familiar with patient's metabolic needs, eating habits, and other lifestyle variables. Inject subQ within 15 minutes before or after a meal.

**Control of hyperglycemia in patients with type 2 diabetes mellitus (Humalog and sulfonyl-ureas)**

■ *Adults and children older than age 3:* Dosage varies and must be determined by prescriber familiar with patient's metabolic needs, eating habits, and other lifestyle variables. Inject subQ within 15 minutes before or after a meal.

## Off-label use

**Hyperkalemia**

■ *Adults:* 50 ml dextrose 50% in water given over 5 minutes, followed by 5 to 10 units of regular insulin by I.V. push.

## Adverse reactions

**Anaphylaxis** • hyperglycemia • hypersensitivity reactions • *hypoglycemia* • hypokalemia • hypo-magnesemia • *lipoatrophy* • *lipohypertrophy* • pruritus • rash • redness • swelling, stinging, urticaria, or warmth at injection site

## Nursing considerations

■ Use only syringes calibrated for the particular concentration of insulin given.

■ Never store U-500 insulin in same area with other insulin preparations because of danger of severe overdose if given accidentally to other patients.

■ To mix insulin suspension, swirl vial gently or rotate between palms. Don't shake vigorously.

■ Lente, semilente, and ultralente insulins may be mixed in any proportion. Regular insulin may be mixed with NPH or lente insulins in any proportion. When mixing regular insulin with intermediate- or long-acting insulin, always draw up regular insulin into syringe first.

■ When NPH or lente is mixed with regular insulin in the same syringe, give immediately.

■ Lispro insulin may be mixed with Humulin N or Humulin U.

■ Don't use insulin that changes color or becomes clumped or granular in appearance.

■ For proper subQ administration, pinch a fold of skin with fingers at least 3 inches (7.6 cm) apart and insert needle at a 45- to 90-degree angle; press but don't rub site after injection. Rotate injection sites to avoid overuse of one area.

## isosorbide
(igh-soh-SOR-bighd)

isosorbide dinitrate
Apo-ISDN†, Cedocard-SR†, Dilatrate-SR, Isordil, Isordil Tembids, Isordil Titradose
isosorbide mononitrate
Imdur, ISMO, Isotrate ER, Monoket

Pregnancy risk category: C

### Indications and dosages

**Acute anginal attacks (S.L. tablets of isosorbide dinitrate only); for prevention in situations likely to cause anginal attacks**
■ *Adults:* 2.5 to 5 mg S.L. tablets for prompt relief of angina, repeated q 5 to 10 minutes (maximum of three doses for each 30-minute period). For prevention, 2.5 to 10 mg q 2 to 3 hours.
■ *Adults:* 5 to 40 mg isosorbide dinitrate P.O. b.i.d. or t.i.d. for prevention only (use smallest effective dose).
■ *Adults:* 30 to 60 mg isosorbide mononitrate (Imdur) P.O. once daily on arising; increase to 120 mg once daily after several days, if needed.
■ *Adults:* 20 mg isosorbide mononitrate (ISMO or Monoket) b.i.d., with the two doses given 7 hours apart.

### Adverse reactions

*Ankle edema* • cutaneous vasodilation • dizziness • fainting • *flushing* • headache • orthostatic hypotension • nausea • *palpitations* • rash • S.L. burning • *tachycardia* • vomiting • weakness

### Nursing considerations

■ Drug is contraindicated in patients with idiosyncratic reactions to nitrates and in those with severe hypotension, shock, or acute MI with low left ventricular filling pressure.

■ To prevent tolerance, a nitrate-free interval of 8 to 12 hours per day is recommended. The regimen for isosorbide mononitrate is intended to minimize nitrate tolerance by providing a substantial nitrate-free interval.

■ Monitor blood pressure and intensity and duration of drug response.

■ Drug may cause headaches, especially at beginning of therapy. Dosage may be reduced temporarily, but tolerance usually develops. Treat headache with aspirin or acetaminophen.

■ Methemoglobinemia has occurred with nitrate use. Signs and symptoms of methemoglobinemia are those of impaired oxygen delivery despite adequate cardiac output and adequate partial pressure of arterial oxygen.

**Watch out!** Don't confuse Isordil with Inderal or Isuprel.

# ketorolac tromethamine
(kee-toh-ROH-lak troh-METH-uh-meen)

Toradol

Pregnancy risk category: C; D in third trimester

## Indications and dosages

### Single-dose treatment of moderately severe, acute pain
■ *Adults younger than age 65:* 60 mg I.M. or 30 mg I.V.
■ *Children ages 2 to 16:* 1 mg/kg I.M. (maximum dosage, 30 mg) or 0.5 mg/kg I.V. (maximum dosage, 15 mg).
■ *Adults age 65 and older:* 30 mg I.M. or 15 mg I.V.
*Adjust-a-dose:* For renally impaired patients or those weighing less than 50 kg (110 lb), 30 mg I.M. or 15 mg I.V.

### Moderately severe, acute pain
■ *Adults younger than age 65:* 30 mg I.M. or I.V. q 6 hours for up to 5 days. Maximum daily dosage, 120 mg.
■ *Adults age 65 and older:* 15 mg I.M. or I.V. q 6 hours for up to 5 days. Maximum dosage, 60 mg daily.
*Adjust-a-dose:* For renally impaired patients or those weighing less than 50 kg, 15 mg I.M. or I.V. q 6 hours. Maximum daily dosage, 60 mg.

### Moderately severe, acute pain when switching to oral therapy
■ *Adults younger than age 65:* 20 mg P.O. as single dose; then 10 mg P.O. q 4 to 6 hours for up to

5 days. Maximum total daily dosage, 40 mg.
■ *Adults age 65 and older:* 10 mg P.O. as single dose; then 10 mg P.O. q 4 to 6 hours for up to 5 days. Maximum daily dosage, 40 mg.
*Adjust-a-dose:* For renally impaired patients or those weighing less than 50 kg, 10 mg P.O. as single dose; then 10 mg P.O. q 4 to 6 hours. Maximum total daily dosage, 40 mg.

## Adverse reactions

Constipation • decreased platelet adhesion • diaphoresis • diarrhea • dizziness • drowsiness • *dyspepsia* • edema • flatulence • *GI pain* • *headache* • hypertension • *nausea* • peptic ulceration • prolonged bleeding time • pruritus • purpura • rash • stomatitis • vomiting

## Nursing considerations

■ Drug is contraindicated in patients with active peptic ulcer disease, recent GI bleeding or perforation, advanced renal impairment, cerebrovascular bleeding, hemorrhagic diathesis, or incomplete hemostasis, and in those at risk for bleeding or renal impairment from volume depletion.

**Watch out!** Don't confuse Toradol with Foradil or Tegretol.

# lamivudine (la-MI-vyoo-deen)

### Epivir, Epivir HBV

Pregnancy risk category: C

## Indications and dosages

### HIV infection (with other anti-retrovirals)

■ *Adults and children older than age 16:* 300 mg Epivir P.O. once daily or 150 mg P.O. b.i.d.
■ *Children ages 3 months to 16 years:* 4 mg/kg Epivir P.O. b.i.d. Maximum dosage, 150 mg b.i.d.

## Off-label use

### HIV infection (with other anti-retrovirals)

*Neonates age 30 days and younger:* 2 mg/kg Epivir P.O. b.i.d.
*Adjust-a-dose:* For patients with creatinine clearance of 30 to 49 ml/minute, give 150 mg Epivir P.O. daily. If clearance is 15 to 29 ml/minute, give 150 mg P.O. on day 1, then 100 mg daily; if 5 to 14 ml/minute, give 150 mg P.O. on day 1, then 50 mg daily; if less than 5 ml/minute, give 50 mg on day 1, then 25 mg daily.

### Chronic hepatitis B with evidence of hepatitis B viral replication and active liver inflammation

■ *Adults:* 100 mg Epivir HBV P.O. once daily.
■ *Children ages 2 to 17:* 3 mg/kg Epivir HBV P.O. once daily, up to a maximum dosage of 100 mg daily.
*Adjust-a-dose:* For adults with creatinine clearance of 30 to 49 ml/minute, give first dose of 100 mg Epivir HBV, then 50 mg P.O. once daily. If clearance is 15 to 29 ml/minute, give first dose of 100 mg, then 25 mg P.O. once daily. If clearance is 5 to 14 ml/minute, give first dose of 35 mg, then 15 mg P.O. once daily. If clearance is less than 5 ml/minute, give first dose of 35 mg, then 10 mg P.O. once daily.

## Adverse reactions

### For combination therapy of lamivudine and zidovudine

Abdominal cramps ▪ abdominal pain ▪ anemia ▪ *anorexia* ▪ arthralgia ▪ *chills* ▪ *cough* ▪ depressive disorders ▪ *diarrhea* ▪ *dizziness* ▪ dyspepsia ▪ *fatigue* ▪ *fever* ▪ *headache* ▪ **hepatotoxicity** ▪ **lactic acidosis** ▪ *malaise* ▪ *musculoskeletal pain* ▪ myalgia ▪ *nasal symptoms* ▪ nausea ▪ neuropathy ▪ **neutropenia** ▪ **pancreatitis** ▪ rash ▪ *sleep disorders* ▪ **thrombocytopenia** ▪ vomiting

## Nursing considerations

*Alert:* Monitor amylase level. Notify prescriber immediately if findings suggest pancreatitis or signs and symptoms of lactic acidosis or hepatotoxicity.
■ Hepatitis may recur in some patients with chronic hepatitis B virus when they stop taking drug.
■ Monitor CBC, platelet count, and kidney and liver function studies. Report abnormalities.

# lansoprazole (lan-SOH-prah-zohl)

Prevacid, Prevacid IV, Prevacid SoluTab

Pregnancy risk category: B

## Indications and dosages

### Active duodenal ulcer
■ *Adults:* 15 mg P.O. daily before eating for 4 weeks. May continue for maintenance treatment

### Active benign gastric ulcer
■ *Adults:* 30 mg P.O. once daily for up to 8 weeks.

### I.V. therapy for erosive esophagitis
■ *Adults:* 30 mg I.V. daily over 30 minutes for up to 7 days. Switch to P.O. form as soon as possible and continue for 6 to 8 weeks.

### Erosive esophagitis
■ *Adults:* 30 mg P.O. daily before eating for up to 16 weeks. Maintenance dosage for healing, 15 mg P.O. daily.
■ *Children ages 12 to 17:* 30 mg P.O. once daily for up to 8 weeks.
■ *Children ages 1 to 11 weighing more than 30 kg (66 lb):* 30 mg P.O. once daily for up to 12 weeks.
■ *Children ages 1 to 11 weighing 30 kg or less:* 15 mg P.O. once daily for up to 12 weeks.

### Pathologic hypersecretory conditions
■ *Adults:* Initially, 60 mg P.O. once daily. Increase dosage, p.r.n. Give daily amounts above 120 mg in evenly divided doses.

### *Helicobacter pylori* eradication to reduce risk of duodenal ulcer recurrence

■ *Adults:* For patients receiving dual therapy, 30 mg P.O. lansoprazole with 1 g P.O. amoxicillin, each given t.i.d. for 14 days. For patients receiving triple therapy, 30 mg P.O. lansoprazole with 1 g P.O. amoxicillin and 500 mg P.O. clarithromycin, all given b.i.d. for 10 to 14 days.

### Symptomatic gastroesophageal reflux disease
■ *Adults:* 15 mg P.O. once daily for up to 8 weeks.
■ *Children ages 12 to 17:* 15 mg P.O. once daily for up to 8 weeks.
■ *Children ages 1 to 11 weighing more than 30 kg:* 30 mg P.O. once daily for up to 12 weeks.
■ *Children ages 1 to 11 weighing 30 kg or less:* 15 mg P.O. once daily for up to 12 weeks.

### NSAID-related ulcer
■ *Adults:* 30 mg P.O. daily for 8 weeks.

### To reduce risk of NSAID-related ulcer in patients with history of gastric ulcer who need NSAIDS
■ *Adults:* 15 mg P.O. daily for up to 12 weeks.

## Adverse reactions
Abdominal pain • diarrhea • nausea

## Nursing considerations
■ Lansoprazole shouldn't be given to breast-feeding women.

126

# lanthanum carbonate
(LAHN-than-uhm KAR-boh-nayt)

Fosrenol

Pregnancy risk category: C

## Indications and dosages

**To reduce serum phosphate level in patients with end-stage renal disease**
■ *Adults:* Initially, 250 to 500 mg P.O. t.i.d. with meals. Adjust every 2 to 3 weeks by 750 mg daily until desired serum phosphate level is reached. Reducing phosphate level to less than 6 mg/dl typically requires 1,500 to 3,000 mg daily.

## Adverse reactions

Abdominal pain ■ bronchitis ■ *constipation* ■ *dialysis graft complications* ■ *dialysis graft occlusion* ■ *diarrhea* ■ headache ■ hypercalcemia ■ *hypotension* ■ *nausea* ■ rhinitis ■ *vomiting*

## Nursing considerations

▢ Give drug with or just after a meal.
▢ Monitor patient for bone pain and skeletal deformities.
▢ Check serum phosphate level during dosage adjustment and regularly p.r.n throughout treatment.
▢ Drug isn't recommended for children because it's deposited in developing bone, including the growth plate.

# latanoprost (lah-TAN-oh-prost)

Xalatan

Pregnancy risk category: C

## Indications and dosages

**First-line treatment of increased intraocular pressure (IOP) in patients with ocular hypertension or open-angle glaucoma**

■ *Adults:* Instill 1 drop in conjunctival sac of affected eye once daily at bedtime.

## Adverse reactions

Allergic skin reactions ● angina pectoris ● *blurred vision* ● *burning and stinging* ● cold ● conjunctival hyperemia ● dry eye ● excessive tearing ● eyelash changes ● eye pain ● flulike syndrome ● *foreign body sensation* ● *increased brown pigmentation of the iris* ● *itching* ● lid crusting or edema ● lid discomfort ● muscle, joint, or back pain ● photophobia ● punctate epithelial keratopathy ● rash ● upper respiratory tract infection

## Nursing considerations

■ Don't give drug while patient is wearing contact lenses.

■ Giving drug more frequently than recommended may decrease its IOP-lowering effects.

■ Drug may gradually change eye color, increasing amount of brown pigment in iris. This change occurs slowly and may not be noticeable for months or years. Increased pigmentation may be permanent.

■ To avoid ocular infections, don't allow tip of dispenser to contact eye or surrounding tissue. Contaminated solutions may cause serious eye damage and subsequent vision loss.

# levofloxacin (lee-voe-FLOX-a-sin)

Levaquin

Pregnancy risk category: C

## Indications and dosages

**Acute maxillary sinusitis**
■ *Adults:* 500 mg P.O. or I.V. daily for 10 to 14 days.

**Mild to moderate skin and skin-structure infections**
■ *Adults:* 500 mg P.O. or I.V. q 24 hours for 7 to 10 days.

**Acute bacterial worsening of chronic bronchitis**
■ *Adults:* 500 mg P.O. or I.V. over 60 minutes q 24 hours for 7 days.

**Community-acquired pneumonia caused by multidrug-resistant Streptococcus pneumoniae (resistance to two or more of the following antibiotics: penicillin, second-generation cephalosporins, macrolides, tetracyclines, tri-methoprim-sulfamethoxazole), Staphylococcus aureus, Moraxella catarrhalis, Haemophilus influenzae, H. parainfluenzae, Klebsiella pneumoniae, Chlamydia pneumoniae, Legionella pneumophila, or Mycoplasma pneumoniae**
■ *Adults:* 500 mg P.O. or I.V. infusion over 60 minutes q 24 hours for 7 to 14 days.

**Chronic bacterial prostatitis**
■ *Adults:* 500 mg P.O. or I.V. over 60 minutes q 24 hours for 28 days.
*Adjust-a-dose:* For patients with creatinine clearance of 20 to 49 ml/minute, give first dose of 500 mg, then 250 mg daily. If clearance is 10 to 19 ml/minute or for patients on dialysis or long-term ambulatory peritoneal dialysis, give first dose of 500 mg, then 250 mg q 48 hours.

**Community-acquired pneumonia caused by S. pneumoniae (excluding multidrug resistant strains), H. influenzae, H. parainfluenzae, M. pneumoniae, and C. pneumoniae**
■ *Adults:* 750 mg P.O. or I.V. over 90 minutes q 24 hours for 5 days.

**Complicated skin and skin-structure infections**
■ *Adults:* 750 mg P.O. or I.V. infusion over 90 minutes q 24 hours for 7 to 14 days.

**Nosocomial pneumonia**
■ *Adults:* 750 mg P.O. or I.V. infusion over 90 minutes q 24 hours for 7 to 14 days.
*Adjust-a-dose:* If creatinine clearance is 20 to 49 ml/minute, give 750 mg initially, then 750 mg q 48 hours; if clearance is 10 to 19 ml/minute, or patient is receiving hemodialysis or long-term ambulatory peritoneal dialysis, give 750 mg initially, then 500 mg q 48 hours.

**Mild to moderate UTI or mild to moderate acute pyelonephritis**
■ *Adults:* 250 mg P.O. or I.V. over 60 minutes q 24 hours for 10 days.
*Adjust-a-dose:* If creatinine clearance is 10 to 19 ml/minute, increase dosage interval to q 48 hours.

*(continued)*

## levofloxacin (continued)

### Mild to moderate uncomplicated UTI
■ *Adults:* 250 mg P.O. daily for 3 days.

### Off-label uses

**Traveler's diarrhea**
■ *Adults:* 500 mg P.O. daily for up to 3 days.
**To prevent traveler's diarrhea**
■ *Adults:* 500 mg P.O. once daily during period of risk, for up to 3 weeks.
**Uncomplicated cervical, urethral, or rectal gonorrhea**
■ *Adults:* 250 mg P.O. as a single dose.

### Adverse reactions

Abdominal pain ▪ allergic pneumonitis ▪ **anaphylaxis** ▪ back pain ▪ chest pain ▪ constipation ▪ diarrhea ▪ dizziness ▪ dyspepsia ▪ **encephalopathy** ▪ eosinophilia ▪ **erythema multiforme** ▪ flatulence ▪ headache ▪ hemolytic anemia ▪ hypersensitivity reactions ▪ **hypoglycemia** ▪ insomnia ▪ **lymphopenia** ▪ **multisystem organ failure** ▪ nausea ▪ pain ▪ palpitations ▪ paresthesia ▪ photosensitivity reactions ▪ pruritus ▪ **pseudomembranous colitis** ▪ rash ▪ **seizures** ▪ **Stevens-Johnson syndrome** ▪ tendon rupture ▪ vaginitis ▪ vasodilation ▪ vomiting

### Nursing considerations

■ Dilute single-dose vial for I.V. administration to 5 mg/ml. Don't infuse other drugs through the same line.
■ Because rapid or bolus delivery may cause hypotension, give by slow I.V. infusion over 60 to 90 minutes.
■ If patient experiences symptoms of excessive CNS stimulation, stop drug and notify prescriber. Begin seizure precautions.
■ Patients with acute hypersensitivity reactions may need treatment with epinephrine, oxygen, I.V. fluids, antihistamines, corticosteroids, pressor amines, or airway management.
■ Most antibacterial drugs, such as levofloxacin, can cause pseudomembranous colitis. Notify prescriber if diarrhea occurs.
■ Obtain specimen for culture and sensitivity testing before starting therapy and p.r.n. to determine if bacterial resistance has occurred.
*Alert:* If *P. aeruginosa* is a confirmed or suspected pathogen, expect to use combination therapy with a beta-lactam.
■ Monitor blood glucose level and renal, hepatic, and hematopoietic blood studies.

# levothyroxine sodium
(lee-voh-thigh-ROKS-een SOH-dee-um)

Eltroxin†, Levo-T, Levothroid, Levoxine, Levoxyl, Synthroid, Thyro-Tabs, Unithroid

Pregnancy risk category: A

## Indications and dosages

**Myxedema coma**
■ *Adults:* 300 to 500 mcg I.V., followed by maintenance dose of 75 to 100 mcg I.V. daily. Switch to oral therapy as soon as possible.
**Thyroid hormone replacement**
■ *Adults:* Initially, 25 to 50 mcg P.O. daily; increase by 25 mcg P.O. q 4 to 8 weeks until desired response occurs. Maintenance dosage, 75 to 200 mcg P.O. daily.
■ *Children older than age 12:* More than 150 mcg or 2 to 3 mcg/kg P.O. daily.
■ *Children ages 6 to 12:* 100 to 150 mcg or 4 to 5 mcg/kg P.O. daily.
■ *Children ages 1 to 5:* 75 to 100 mcg or 5 to 6 mcg/kg P.O. daily.
■ *Children ages 6 months to 1 year:* 50 to 75 mcg or 6 to 8 mcg/kg P.O. daily.
■ *Children younger than age 6 months:* 25 to 50 mcg or 8 to 10 mcg/kg P.O. daily.
■ *Adults older than age 65:* 12.5 to 50 mcg P.O. daily; increase by 12.5 to 25 mcg q 6 to 8 weeks, depending on response.

## Adverse reactions

Allergic skin reactions • *angina pectoris* • **arrhythmias** • **cardiac arrest** • decreased bone density • diaphoresis • diarrhea • fever • headache • heat intolerance • *insomnia* • menstrual irregularities • *nervousness* • *palpitations* • *tachycardia* • *tremor* • vomiting • weight loss

## Nursing considerations

■ Patients with diabetes mellitus may need increased antidiabetic dosages when starting thyroid hormone replacement.
■ Observe patients with coronary artery disease carefully for possible coronary insufficiency.
■ Patients with adult hypothyroidism are unusually sensitive to thyroid hormone. Monitor closely.
■ When changing from levothyroxine to liothyronine, stop levothyroxine and begin liothyronine. Increase dosage in small increments, as prescribed, after residual effects of levothyroxine have disappeared. When changing from liothyronine to levothyroxine, start levothyroxine several days before withdrawing liothyronine to avoid relapse. Drugs aren't interchangeable.
■ Stop drug 4 weeks before [131]I uptake studies.
**Watch out!** Don't confuse levothyroxine with liothyronine or liotrix.

# lisinopril (ligh-SIN-uh-pril)

Prinivil, Zestril

Pregnancy risk category: C; D in second and third trimesters

## Indications and dosages

### Hypertension

■ *Adults:* Initially, 10 mg P.O. daily for patients not taking a diuretic. Usual range, 20 to 40 mg daily as a single dose. For patients taking a diuretic, initially, 5 mg P.O. daily.

*Adjust-a-dose:* If creatinine clearance is 10 to 30 ml/minute, give 5 mg P.O. daily; if clearance is less than 10 ml/minute, give 2.5 mg P.O. daily.

### Heart failure (with diuretics and cardiac glycosides)

■ *Adults:* Initially, 5 mg P.O. daily; increased, p.r.n., to maximum of 20 mg P.O. daily.

*Adjust-a-dose:* If sodium level is less than 130 mEq/L or creatinine clearance is less than 30 ml/minute, start treatment at 2.5 mg daily.

### Hemodynamically stable patients within 24 hours of acute MI to improve survival

■ *Adults:* Initially, 5 mg P.O.; then 5 mg after 24 hours, 10 mg after 48 hours, followed by 10 mg once daily for 6 weeks.

*Adjust-a-dose:* For patients with systolic blood pressure of 120 mm Hg or less at start of treatment or during first 3 days after an infarct, decrease dosage to 2.5 mg P.O. If systolic blood pressure drops to 100 mm Hg or less, reduce daily maintenance dosage of 5 mg to

2.5 mg. If systolic blood pressure remains below 90 mm Hg for longer than 1 hour, stop drug.

### Hypertension in children

■ *Children ages 6 to 16:* Initially, 0.07 mg/kg P.O. once daily (up to 5 mg total), then adjust accordingly.

## Adverse reactions

Chest pain • *diarrhea* • *dizziness* • dry, persistent, tickling, nonproductive cough • dyspepsia • dyspnea • fatigue • headache • *hyperkalemia* • hypotension • impaired renal function • impotence • nausea • *orthostatic hypotension* • *nasal congestion* paresthesia • rash

## Nursing considerations

■ Black patients should take drug with a thiazide diuretic for a more favorable response.
■ ACE inhibitors appear to increase the risk of angioedema in black patients.
■ Monitor blood pressure frequently.
■ Monitor WBC with differential counts before therapy, every 2 weeks for first 3 months of therapy, and periodically thereafter.

**Watch out!** Don't confuse lisinopril with fosinopril or Lioresal. Don't confuse Prinivil with Prilosec or Proventil. Don't confuse Zestril with Zebeta, Zetia, Zostrix, or Zyrtec.

# loperamide (loh-PEH-ruh-mighd)

Imodium, Imodium A-D, Kaopectate II Caplets, Maalox Anti-Diarrheal Caplets, Pepto Diarrhea Control

Pregnancy risk category: **B**

## Indications and dosages

**Acute, nonspecific diarrhea**
■ *Adults and children older than age 12:* Initially, 4 mg P.O.; then 2 mg after each unformed stool. Maximum dosage, 8 mg daily unless otherwise directed.
■ *Children ages 8 to 12:* 2 mg P.O. t.i.d. on first day. Subsequent dosages of 5 ml or 0.1 mg/kg of body weight may be given after each unformed stool. Maximum dosage, 6 mg daily.
■ *Children ages 6 to 8:* 2 mg P.O. b.i.d. on first day. If diarrhea persists, contact prescriber. Maximum dosage, 4 mg daily.
■ *Children ages 2 to 5:* 1 mg P.O. t.i.d. on first day. If diarrhea persists, contact prescriber.

**Chronic diarrhea**
■ *Adults:* Initially, 4 mg P.O.; then 2 mg after each unformed stool until diarrhea subsides. Adjust dosage to individual response.

## Adverse reactions

Abdominal pain, distention, or discomfort • *constipation* • dizziness • drowsiness • dry mouth • fatigue • hypersensitivity reactions • nausea • rash • vomiting

## Nursing considerations

*Alert:* Monitor children closely for CNS effects; children may be more sensitive to these effects than adults are.
■ If clinical symptoms don't improve within 48 hours, stop therapy and notify prescriber.
■ Drug produces antidiarrheal action similar to that of diphenoxylate but without as many adverse CNS effects.
**Watch out!** Don't confuse Imodium with Ionamin.

# loratadine (loo-RAH-tuh-deen)

Alavert, Claritin, Claritin Reditabs, Claritin Syrup, Tavist ND Allergy

Pregnancy risk category: B

## Indications and dosages

**Hay fever or other upper respiratory allergies; chronic idiopathic urticaria**

■ *Adults and children age 6 and older:* 10 mg P.O. daily.
■ *Children ages 2 to 5:* 5 mg P.O. daily.

*Adjust-a-dose:* For adults and children ages 6 and older with hepatic failure or creatinine clearance less than 30 ml/minute, adjust dosage to 10 mg every other day. For children ages 2 to 5 with hepatic failure or renal insufficiency, adjust dosage to 5 mg every other day.

## Adverse reactions

Drowsiness • dry mouth • fatigue • *headache* • insomnia • nervousness

## Nursing considerations

■ Drug should be stopped 4 days before patient undergoes diagnostic skin tests because drug can prevent, reduce, or mask positive skin test response.

## lorazepam (loo-RAZ-eh-pam)

Apo-Lorazepam†, Ativan, Lorazepam Intensol, Novo-Lorazem†, Nu-Loraz†

Pregnancy risk category: **D**

### Indications and dosages

**Anxiety**
■ *Adults:* 2 to 6 mg P.O. daily in divided doses. Maximum dosage, 10 mg daily.
■ *Elderly patients:* 1 to 2 mg P.O. daily in divided doses. Maximum dosage, 10 mg daily.

**Insomnia from anxiety**
■ *Adults:* 2 to 4 mg P.O. at bedtime.

**Preoperative sedation**
■ *Adults:* 0.05 mg/kg I.M. 2 hours before procedure. Total dose should not exceed 4 mg. Or, 2 mg I.V. total or 0.044 mg/kg I.V., whichever is smaller. Larger doses up to 0.05 mg/kg I.V., to a total of 4 mg, may be needed.

### Off-label uses

**Status epilepticus**
■ *Adults and children:* 0.05 to 0.1 mg/kg. Repeat q 10 to 15 minutes, p.r.n. Or, give adults 4 to 8 mg I.V.

**Nausea and vomiting caused by emetogenic cancer chemotherapy**
■ *Adults:* 2.5 mg P.O. the evening before and just after starting chemotherapy. Or, 1.5 mg/m$^2$ (usually up to a maximum of 3 mg) I.V. over 5 minutes, 45 minutes before starting chemotherapy.

### Adverse reactions

Abdominal discomfort ● agitation ● amnesia ● change in appetite ● depression ● disorientation ● dizziness ● *drowsiness* ● headache ● hypotension ● insomnia ● nausea ● *sedation* ● unsteadiness ● vision disturbances ● weakness

### Nursing considerations

■ Drug is contraindicated in patients with angle-closure glaucoma and in patients hypersensitive to benzodiazepines or the vehicle used in parenteral forms.
***Alert:*** Use of this drug may lead to abuse and addiction. Drug shouldn't be stopped abruptly after long-term use because withdrawal symptoms may occur.
■ For I.V. use, dilute lorazepam with an equal volume of compatible diluent, such as D$_5$W, sterile water for injection, or normal saline solution. The rate of I.V. injection shouldn't exceed 2 mg/minute. Keep emergency resuscitative equipment readily available.
■ For I.M. administration, inject deeply into muscle. Don't dilute.
■ Refrigerate parenteral form to prolong shelf life.
■ Monitor hepatic, renal, and hematopoietic function periodically in patients receiving repeated or prolonged therapy.
**Watch out!** Don't confuse lorazepam with alprazolam.

I.M.

# losartan potassium (loh-SAR-tan poh-TAH-see-um)

Cozaar

Pregnancy risk category: C; D in second and third trimesters

## Indications and dosages

**Hypertension**

■ *Adults:* Initially, 25 to 50 mg P.O. daily. Maximum dosage, 100 mg daily in one or two divided doses. *Adjust-a-dose:* For patients who are hepatically impaired or intravascularly volume-depleted (such as those taking diuretics), initially, 25 mg.

**Nephropathy in patients with type 2 diabetes mellitus**

■ *Adults:* 50 mg P.O. once daily. Increase dosage to 100 mg once daily based on blood pressure response.

**To reduce risk of stroke in patients with hypertension and left ventricular hypertrophy**

■ *Adults:* Initially, 50 mg losartan P.O. once daily. Adjust dosage based on blood pressure response, adding hydrochlorothiazide 12.5 mg once daily, increasing losartan to 100 mg daily, or both. If further adjustments are needed, may increase the daily dosage of hydrochlorothiazide to 25 mg.

## Adverse reactions

**Patients with hypertension or left ventricular hypertrophy**
Abdominal pain ▪ *angioedema* ▪ asthenia ▪ back or leg pain ▪ chest pain ▪ cough ▪ diarrhea ▪ dizziness ▪ dyspepsia ▪ edema ▪ fatigue ▪ headache ▪ insomnia ▪ muscle cramps ▪ myalgia ▪ nasal congestion ▪ nausea ▪ pharyngitis ▪ sinus disorder ▪ sinusitis ▪ upper respiratory tract infection

**Patients with nephropathy**
Anemia ▪ *angioedema* ▪ asthenia ▪ back pain ▪ cataract ▪ bronchitis ▪ chest pain ▪ cough ▪ diabetic neuropathy ▪ *diabetic vascular disease* ▪ diarrhea ▪ dyspepsia ▪ fatigue ▪ fever ▪ flulike syndrome ▪ gastritis ▪ *hyperkalemia* ▪ hypoesthesia ▪ *hypoglycemia* ▪ hypotension ▪ infection ▪ leg or knee pain ▪ muscle weakness ▪ orthostatic hypotension ▪ sinusitis ▪ trauma ▪ *UTI* ▪ weight gain

## Nursing considerations

■ Drug can be used alone or with other antihypertensives.
■ Monitor patient's blood pressure closely to evaluate effectiveness of therapy. When used alone, drug has less of an effect on blood pressure in black patients than in patients of other races.
■ Watch for symptomatic hypotension in patients who are also taking diuretics.
■ Regularly assess the patient's renal function (via creatinine and BUN levels).
**Watch out!** Don't confuse Cozaar with Zocor.

# magnesium sulfate (mag-NEE-see-um SUL-fayt)

Pregnancy risk category: A

## Indications and dosages

**To prevent or control seizures in preeclampsia or eclampsia**
■ *Women:* Initially, 4 g I.V. in 250 ml $D_5W$ or normal saline solution and 4 to 5 g deep I.M. into each buttock; then 4 to 5 g deep I.M. into alternate buttock q 4 hours, p.r.n. Or, 4 g I.V. loading dose; then 1 to 3 g hourly as I.V. infusion. Total dose shouldn't exceed 30 or 40 g daily.

**Hypomagnesemia**
■ *Adults:* For mild deficiency, 1 g I.M. q 6 hours for four doses; for severe deficiency, 5 g in 1,000 ml $D_5W$ or normal saline solution infused over 3 hours.

**Seizures, hypertension, and encephalopathy with acute nephritis in children**
■ *Children:* 0.2 ml/kg of 50% solution I.M. q 4 to 6 hours, p.r.n. For severe symptoms, 100 to 200 mg/kg as a 1% to 3% solution I.V. slowly over 1 hour with 50% of dose given in first 15 to 20 minutes. Adjust dosage according to magnesium level and seizure response.

**Paroxysmal atrial tachycardia**
■ *Adults:* 3 to 4 g I.V. over 30 seconds, with extreme caution.

## Off-label uses

**Life-threatening ventricular arrhythmias**
■ *Adults:* 1 to 6 g I.V. over several minutes; then continuous I.V. infusion of 3 to 20 mg/minute for 5 to 48 hours.
■ *Adults:* 4 to 6 g I.V. over 20 minutes, followed by 2 to 4 g/hour I.V. infusion for 12 to 24 hours, as tolerated, after contractions have ceased.

## Adverse reactions

**Bradycardia** • *circulatory collapse* • depressed cardiac function • *depressed reflexes* • diaphoresis • diplopia • drowsiness • flaccid paralysis • *flushing* • hypocalcemia • *hypotension* • hypothermia • **respiratory paralysis**

## Nursing considerations

■ Parenteral use is contraindicated in patients with heart block or myocardial damage.
**Alert:** Watch for respiratory depression and heart block.
■ Keep I.V. calcium gluconate available to reverse magnesium intoxication, but use cautiously in digitalized patients.
■ Disappearance of knee-jerk and patellar reflexes is a sign of impending magnesium toxicity.
■ Make sure urine output is 100 ml or more in 4-hour period before each dose.
■ Observe neonate for signs and symptoms of magnesium toxicity, including respiratory depression, if given within 24 hours of birth.
**Watch out!** Don't confuse magnesium with manganese.

# mannitol (MAN-ih-tol)

Osmitrol

Pregnancy risk category: C

## Indications and dosages

**Test dose for marked oliguria or suspected inadequate renal function**

■ *Adults and children older than age 12:* 200 mg/kg or 12.5 g as a 15% to 20% I.V. solution over 3 to 5 minutes. Response is adequate if 30 to 50 ml of urine/hour is excreted over 2 to 3 hours; if response is inadequate, repeat.

**Oliguria**

■ *Adults and children older than age 12:* 50 to 100 g I.V. as a 15% to 25% solution over 90 minutes to several hours.

**To prevent oliguria or acute renal failure**

■ *Adults and children older than age 12:* 50 to 100 g I.V. of a 5% to 25% solution. Determine exact concentration by fluid requirements.

**To reduce intraocular or intracranial pressure**

■ *Adults and children older than age 12:* 1.5 to 2 g/kg as a 15% to 20% I.V. solution over 30 to 60 minutes. For maximum intraocular pressure reduction before surgery, give 60 to 90 minutes preoperatively.

**Diuresis in drug intoxication**

■ *Adults and children older than age 12:* 5% to 10% solution continuously up to 200 g I.V., while maintaining 100 to 500 ml urine output/ hour and a positive fluid balance.

## Adverse reactions

Angina-like chest pain ▪ blurred vision ▪ chills ▪ dehydration ▪ *diarrhea* ▪ dizziness ▪ dry mouth ▪ edema ▪ fever ▪ headache ▪ *heart failure* ▪ hypertension ▪ hypotension ▪ local pain ▪ nausea ▪ rhinitis ▪ *seizures* ▪ tachycardia ▪ thirst ▪ thrombophlebitis ▪ urine retention ▪ urticaria ▪ vascular overload ▪ vomiting

## Nursing considerations

■ Drug is contraindicated in patients with anuria, severe pulmonary edema, severe heart failure, severe dehydration, metabolic edema, progressive renal disease, and active intracranial bleeding (except during craniotomy).

■ Give drug I.V. via an in-line filter and avoid extravasation.

■ Monitor vital signs and central venous pressure and fluid intake and output, hourly. Report increasing oliguria. Check weight, renal function, fluid balance, and serum and urine sodium and potassium levels daily.

■ Use urinary catheter in comatose or incontinent patient for strict evaluation of fluid intake and output.

## metformin hydrochloride
(met-FOR-min high-droh-KLOR-ighd)

Fortamet, Glucophage, Glucophage XR, Riomet

Pregnancy risk category: **B**

### Indications and dosages

**Adjunct to diet in patients with type 2 diabetes mellitus**

■ *Adults:* For regular-release tablets or oral solution, initially 500 mg P.O. b.i.d. with morning and evening meals, or 850 mg P.O. once daily with morning meal. When 500-mg dose is used, increase dosage by 500 mg weekly to maximum of 2,500 mg P.O. daily in divided doses, p.r.n. When 850-mg dose is used, increase dosage by 850 mg every other week to maximum of 2,550 mg P.O. daily in divided doses, p.r.n. For extended-release formulation, start therapy at 500 mg P.O. once daily with evening meal. May increase dosage weekly in increments of 500 mg daily to maximum of 2,000 mg once daily.

■ *Children ages 10 to 16:* 500 mg P.O. b.i.d. (regular-release form only). Increase dosage in increments of 500 mg weekly to maximum of 2,000 mg daily in divided doses.

*Adjust-a-dose:* For debilitated or elderly patients, dosing should be conservative because of potential decrease in renal function.

**Adjunct to diet and exercise in type 2 diabetes as monotherapy or with a sulfonylurea or insulin (Fortamet)**

■ *Adults age 17 and older:* Initially, 500 to 1,000 mg P.O. with evening meal. Increase dosage based on glucose level in increments of 500 mg weekly to maximum of 2,500 mg daily. When used with a sulfonylurea or insulin, base dosage on glucose level and adjust slowly until desired therapeutic effect occurs. Decrease insulin dosage by 10% to 25% when fasting blood glucose level is less than 120 mg/dl.

*Adjust-a-dose:* For elderly, malnourished, or debilitated patients, don't titrate to maximum dosage.

### Adverse reactions

Abdominal bloating ▪ anorexia ▪ diarrhea ▪ flatulence ▪ ***lactic acidosis*** ▪ megaloblastic anemia ▪ nausea ▪ taste perversion ▪ vomiting

### Nursing considerations

■ Assess patient's renal function before therapy and annually thereafter.

*Alert:* Notify prescriber if patient develops hypoxemia or dehydration because of risk of lactic acidosis.

■ Monitor patient's blood glucose level regularly.

■ Monitor patient closely during times of increased stress. Insulin therapy may be needed.

**Watch out!** Don't confuse Glucophage with Glucovance.

# methylphenidate hydrochloride
(meth-il-FEN-ih-dayt high-droh-KLOR-ighd)

Concerta, Metadate CD, Metadate ER, Methylin, Methylin ER, Ritalin, Ritalin LA, Ritalin-SR

Pregnancy risk category: **NR; C**
(Concerta, Metadate CD, Ritalin LA)

## Indications and dosages

**Attention deficit hyperactivity disorder (ADHD)**

■ *Children age 6 and older:* Initially, 5 mg P.O. b.i.d. immediate-release form before breakfast and lunch, increasing by 5 to 10 mg weekly, p.r.n., until an optimum daily dosage of 2 mg/kg is reached, not to exceed 60 mg/day. To use Ritalin-SR, Metadate ER, and Methylin ER tablets in place of immediate-release methylphenidate tablets, calculate methylphenidate dosage in 8-hour intervals.

*Concerta*

■ *Children age 6 and older not currently taking methylphenidate or patients taking stimulants other than methylphenidate:* 18 mg P.O. (extended-release) once daily q morning. Adjust dosage by 18 mg weekly to a maximum of 54 mg daily q morning.

■ *Children age 6 and older currently taking methylphenidate:* If previous methylphenidate dosage was 5 mg b.i.d. or t.i.d. or 20 mg sustained-release, give 18 mg P.O. q morning. If previous methylphenidate dosage was 10 mg b.i.d. or t.i.d. or 40 mg sustained-release, give 36 mg P.O. q morning. If previous methylphen-

idate dosage was 15 mg b.i.d. or t.i.d. or 60 mg sustained-release, give 54 mg P.O. q morning. Maximum dosage, 54 mg daily.

*Metadate CD*

■ *Children ages 6 and older:* Initially, 20 mg P.O. daily before breakfast, increasing by 20 mg at weekly intervals to maximum of 60 mg daily.

*Ritalin LA*

■ *Children age 6 and older:* 20 mg P.O. once daily. Increase by 10 mg at weekly intervals to maximum of 60 mg daily. If previous methylphenidate dosage was 10 mg b.i.d. or 20 mg sustained-release, give 20 mg P.O. once daily. If previous methylphenidate dosage was 15 mg b.i.d., give 30 mg P.O. once daily. If previous methylphenidate dosage was 20 mg b.i.d. or 40 mg sustained-release, give 40 mg P.O. once daily. If previous methylphenidate dosage was 30 mg b.i.d. or 60 mg sustained-release, give 60 mg P.O. once daily.

**Narcolepsy**

■ *Adults:* 10 mg P.O. b.i.d. or t.i.d. immediate-release form, 30 to 45 minutes before meals. Average dosage, 40 to 60 mg/day. To use Ritalin-SR, Metadate ER, or Methylin ER tablets in place of immediate-release methylphenidate tablets, calculate the dose of methylphenidate in 8-hour intervals.

## methylphenidate hydrochloride *(continued)*

### Adverse reactions

Abdominal pain ▪ akathisia ▪ anemia ▪ anorexia ▪ **arrhythmias** ▪ cough ▪ dizziness ▪ drowsiness ▪ dyskinesia ▪ **erythema multiforme** ▪ *exfoliative dermatitis* ▪ *headache* ▪ hypertension ▪ *insomnia* ▪ **leukopenia** ▪ nausea ▪ *nervousness* ▪ *palpitations* ▪ pharyngitis ▪ rash ▪ **seizures** ▪ sinusitis ▪ *tachycardia* ▪ **thrombocytopenia** ▪ tics ▪ upper respiratory tract infection ▪ urticaria ▪ vomiting ▪ weight loss

### Nursing considerations

▪ Drug is contraindicated in patients with glaucoma, motor tics, a family history of Tourette syndrome, or a history of marked anxiety, tension, or agitation.

▪ Concerta is contraindicated in patients with severe GI narrowing, or within 14 days after taking an MAO inhibitor.

▪ Periodically monitor CBC with differential and platelet counts in patients on long-term therapy.

▪ Monitor height and weight in children; drug may delay growth.

▪ Monitor patient for tolerance or psychological dependence.

**Watch out!** Don't confuse Ritalin with Rifadin.

# methylprednisolone (meth-il-pred-NIS-uh-lohn)

methylprednisolone
**Medrol**
methylprednisolone acetate
**depMedalone 40, depMedalone 80, Depo-Medrol, Depopred-40, Depopred-80**
methylprednisolone sodium succinate
**A-Methapred, Solu-Medrol**

Pregnancy risk category: C

## Indications and dosages

### Severe inflammation or immuno-suppression

■ *Adults:* 2 to 60 mg base P.O. usually in four divided doses, or 10 to 80 mg acetate I.M. daily, or 10 to 250 mg succinate I.M. or I.V. up to six times daily. Or, 4 to 40 mg acetate into smaller joints or 20 to 80 mg acetate into larger joints. Intralesional use is usually 20 to 60 mg acetate. Intralesional and intra-articular injections may be repeated q 1 to 5 weeks.
■ *Children:* 0.03 to 0.2 mg/kg or 1 to 6.25 mg/m$^2$ succinate I.M. once daily or b.i.d.

### Shock

■ *Adults:* 100 to 250 mg succinate I.V. at 2- to 6-hour intervals. Or, 30 mg/kg I.V. initially, repeated q 4 to 6 hours, p.r.n. Give over 3 to 15 minutes. Continue therapy for 2 to 3 days or until patient is stable.

## Adverse reactions

Acne ● *acute adrenal insufficiency with increased stress or following abrupt withdrawal after long-term therapy* ● arrhythmias ● *cardiac arrest* ● *circulatory collapse* ● cushingoid state ● delayed wound healing ● edema ● *euphoria* ● GI irritation ● glaucoma ● growth suppression ● headache ● *heart failure* ● hirsutism ● hypercholesterolemia ● hyperglycemia ● hypertension ● hypocalcemia ● hypokalemia ● increased appetite ● *insomnia* ● menstrual irregularities ● muscle weakness ● nausea ● osteoporosis ● *pancreatitis* ● paresthesia ● *peptic ulceration* ● *pseudotumor cerebri* ● psychotic behavior ● *seizures* ● susceptibility to infections ● *thromboembolism* ● thrombophlebitis ● skin eruptions ● vertigo ● vomiting

## Nursing considerations

■ Drug is contraindicated in patients with systemic fungal infections and in premature infants (acetate and succinate).
*Alert:* Sudden withdrawal after prolonged use may be fatal.
*Alert:* Salt formulations aren't interchangeable.
■ Watch for depression or psychotic episodes.
■ **Watch out!** Don't confuse methylprednisolone with medroxyprogesterone. Don't confuse Solu-Medrol with Solu-Cortef.

# metoprolol (meh-TOH-pruh-lol)

metoprolol succinate
Toprol-XL
metoprolol tartrate
Apo-Metoprolol†, Apo-Metoprolol (Type L)†, Betaloc Durules†, Lopresor†, Lopresor SR†, Lopressor, Novo-Metoprol†, Nu-Metop†

Pregnancy risk category: C

## Indications and dosages

### Hypertension
■ *Adults:* Initially, 50 mg P.O. b.i.d. or 100 mg P.O. once daily; then up to 100 to 450 mg daily in two or three divided doses. Or, 50 to 100 mg extended-release tablets (tartrate equivalent) once daily. Adjust dosage weekly to maximum of 400 mg daily.

### Early intervention in acute MI
■ *Adults:* 5 mg metoprolol tartrate I.V. bolus q 2 minutes for three doses. Then, 15 minutes after the last I.V. dose, give 25 to 50 mg P.O. q 6 hours for 48 hours. Maintenance dosage, 100 mg P.O. b.i.d.

### Angina pectoris
■ *Adults:* Initially, 100 mg P.O. daily as single dose or in two equally divided doses; increased weekly until adequate response or maximum dosage of 400 mg is reached. Or, 100 mg extended-release tablets (tartrate equivalent) once daily. Adjust dosage weekly to maximum of 400 mg daily.

### Stable, symptomatic heart failure (New York Heart Association class II) resulting from ischemia, hypertension, or cardiomyopathy
■ *Adults:* 25 mg (Toprol-XL) P.O. once daily for 2 weeks. Double the dosage q 2 weeks, as tolerated, to maximum of 200 mg daily.
*Adjust-a-dose:* For patients with more severe heart failure, start with 12.5 mg (Toprol-XL) P.O. once daily.

## Adverse reactions

*AV block* • *bradycardia* • diarrhea • depression • *dizziness* • *fatigue* • dyspnea • *heart failure* • hypotension • nausea • rash

## Nursing considerations

■ When used to treat hypertension or angina, contraindicated in patients with bradycardia, greater than first-degree heart block, cardiogenic shock, or overt cardiac failure. When used to treat MI, contraindicated in patients with heart rate less than 45 beats/minute, greater than first-degree heart block, PR interval of 0.24 second or longer with first-degree heart block, systolic blood pressure less than 100 mm Hg, or moderate to severe cardiac failure.

■ Check apical pulse before giving drug. Withhold drug and notify prescriber if pulse is less than 60 beats/minute.

**Watch out!** Don't confuse metoprolol with metaproterenol or metolazone. Don't confuse Toprol with Topamax.

# metronidazole (met-roh-NIGH-duh-zohl)

Apo-Metronidazole†, Flagyl, Flagyl 375, Flagyl ER, Novo-Nidazol†, Protostat, Trikacide†
metronidazole hydrochloride
Flagyl IV RTU, Novonidazol†

Pregnancy risk category: B

## Indications and dosages

### Amebic liver abscess
■ *Adults:* 500 to 750 mg P.O. t.i.d. for 5 to 10 days, or 2.4 g P.O. once daily for 1 to 2 days. Or, 500 mg I.V. q 6 hours for 10 days.
■ *Children:* 30 to 50 mg/kg P.O. daily in three divided doses for 10 days. Maximum dosage, 750 mg/dose.

### Intestinal amebiasis
■ *Adults:* 750 mg P.O. t.i.d. for 5 to 10 days.
■ *Children:* 30 to 50 mg/kg P.O. daily in three divided doses for 10 days.

### Trichomoniasis
■ *Adults:* 250 mg P.O. t.i.d. for 7 days, or 500 mg P.O. b.i.d. for 7 days, or 2 g P.O. in single dose; 4 to 6 weeks should elapse before repeat courses of therapy are given.
■ *Children:* 5 mg/kg P.O. t.i.d. for 7 days.

### Refractory trichomoniasis
■ *Adults:* 250 mg P.O. b.i.d. for 10 days. Or, 500 mg P.O. b.i.d. for 7 days.

### Bacterial infections caused by anaerobic microorganisms
■ *Adults:* Loading dose, 15 mg/kg I.V. over 1 hour, then 7.5 mg/kg I.V. or P.O. q 6 hours, starting 6 hours after loading dose. Maximum dosage, 4 g daily.

### To prevent postoperative infection in contaminated or potentially contaminated colorectal surgery
■ *Adults:* 15 mg/kg I.V. infused over 30 to 60 minutes and completed about 1 hour before surgery. Then, 7.5 mg/kg I.V. infused over 30 to 60 minutes at 6 and 12 hours after first dose.

### Bacterial vaginosis
■ *Adults:* 750 mg (Flagyl ER) P.O. daily for 7 days.

## Adverse reactions

Candidiasis ● confusion ● depression ● diarrhea ● dizziness ● dry mouth ● edema ● epigastric distress ● fever ● flattened T wave ● joint pains ● flushing ● *headache* ● incoordination ● insomnia ● irritability ● metallic taste ● *nausea* ● **neutropenia** ● overgrowth of non-susceptible organisms ● peripheral neuropathy ● rash ● **seizures** ● **transient leukopenia** ● vaginitis ● vertigo ● vomiting ● weakness

## Nursing considerations

■ Monitor liver function test results carefully in elderly patients.
■ Infuse I.V. form over 30 minutes to 1 hour. Don't give I.V. push.
■ Give oral form with meals.

## midazolam hydrochloride
(MID-ayz-oh-lam high-droh-KLOR-ighd)

**Versed, Versed Syrup**

Pregnancy risk category: **D**

### Indications and dosages

**Preoperative sedation**
- *Adults:* 0.07 to 0.08 mg/kg I.M. about 1 hour before surgery.

**Conscious sedation before short procedures**
- *Adults younger than age 60:* Initially, small dose not to exceed 2.5 mg I.V. given slowly; repeat in 2 minutes, if needed, in small increments of first dose over at least 2 minutes to achieve desired effect. Total dose of up to 5 mg may be used. Additional doses to maintain desired level of sedation may be given by slow titration in increments of 25% of dose used to first reach the sedative end point.
- *Patients age 60 and older and debilitated patients:* 0.5 to 1.5 mg I.V. over at least 2 minutes. Incremental doses shouldn't exceed 1 mg. A total dose of up to 3.5 mg is usually sufficient.

**Preoperative or preprocedural in children**

*P.O.*
- *Children ages 6 to 16 and cooperative patients:* 0.25 to 0.5 mg/kg P.O. as a single dose, up to 20 mg.
- *Infants and children ages 6 months to 5 years and less-cooperative patients:* 0.25 to 1 mg/kg P.O. as a single dose, up to 20 mg.

*I.V.*
- *Children ages 12 to 16:* Initially, no more than 2.5 mg I.V. given slowly; repeat in 2 minutes, if needed, in small increments of first dose over at least 2 minutes. Total dose of up to 10 mg may be used. Additional doses may be given by increments of 25% of dose used to first reach the sedative end point.
- *Children ages 6 to 12:* 0.025 to 0.05 mg/kg I.V. over 2 to 3 minutes. Additional doses may be given in small increments after 2 to 3 minutes. Total dose of up to 0.4 mg/kg, not to exceed 10 mg, may be used.
- *Children ages 6 months to 5 years:* 0.05 to 0.1 mg/kg I.V. over 2 to 3 minutes. Additional doses may be given in small increments after 2 to 3 minutes. Total dose of up to 0.6 mg/kg, not to exceed 6 mg, may be used.

*I.M.*
- *Children:* 0.1 to 0.15 mg/kg I.M. Use up to 0.5 mg/kg in more anxious patients.
*Adjust-a-dose:* For obese children, base dosage on ideal body weight; high-risk or debilitated children and children receiving other sedatives need lower dosages.

*(continued)*

## midazolam hydrochloride (continued)

### To induce general anesthesia

■ *Adults older than age 55:* 0.3 mg/kg I.V. over 20 to 30 seconds if patient hasn't received premedication, or 0.2 mg/kg I.V. over 20 to 30 seconds if patient has received a sedative or opioid premedication. Additional increments of 25% of first dose may be needed to complete induction.

■ *Adults younger than age 55:* 0.3 to 0.35 mg/kg I.V. over 20 to 30 seconds if patient hasn't received premedication, or 0.25 mg/kg I.V. over 20 to 30 seconds if patient has received a sedative or opioid premedication. Additional increments of 25% of first dose may be needed to complete induction.

*Adjust-a-dose:* For debilitated patients, initially, 0.2 to 0.25 mg/kg. As little as 0.15 mg/kg may be needed.

### Sedation for intubated patients in critical care unit

■ *Adults:* Initially, 0.01 to 0.05 mg/kg may be given I.V. over several minutes, repeated at 10- to 15-minute intervals as needed until adequate sedation is achieved. Then start continuous infusion at 0.02 to 0.1 mg/kg/hour. Higher loading dose or infusion rates may be needed in some patients.

■ *Children:* Initially, 0.05 to 0.2 mg/kg may be given I.V. over 2 to 3 minutes or longer; then start continuous infusion at a rate of 0.06 to 0.12 mg/kg/hour. Increase or decrease infusion to maintain desired effect.

■ *Neonates more than 32 weeks' gestational age:* Initially, 0.06 mg/kg/hour. Adjust rate p.r.n.

■ *Neonates less than 32 weeks' gestational age:* Initially, 0.03 mg/kg/hour. Adjust rate p.r.n. using lowest possible rate.

### Adverse reactions

**APNEA** • amnesia • *blood pressure* and pulse *variations* • *decreased respiratory rate* • *drowsiness* • headache • hiccups • involuntary movements • *nausea* • nystagmus • *oversedation* • *pain at injection site* • paradoxical excitement • vomiting

### Nursing considerations

■ Drug is contraindicated in patients with angle-closure glaucoma, and those in shock, coma, or acute alcohol intoxication.

*Alert:* Before giving drug, have oxygen and resuscitation equipment available. Excessive amounts and rapid infusion can cause respiratory arrest.

■ When injecting I.M., give deeply into large muscle.

■ Monitor blood pressure, heart rate and rhythm, respirations, airway integrity, and arterial oxygen saturation during procedure.

**Watch out!** Don't confuse Versed with VePesid.

## montelukast sodium
(mon-tih-LOO-kist SOH-dee-um)

Singulair

Pregnancy risk category: **B**

### Indications and dosages

**Asthma, seasonal allergic rhinitis**
■ *Adults and children age 15 and older:* 10 mg P.O. once daily in evening.
■ *Children ages 6 to 14:* 5 mg (chewable tablet) P.O. once daily in evening.
■ *Children ages 2 to 5:* 4 mg chewable tablet or 1 packet of oral granules P.O. once daily in the evening.
■ *Children ages 12 to 23 months (asthma only):* 1 packet of oral granules P.O. once daily in the evening.

### Adverse reactions

Abdominal pain ▪ asthenia ▪ cough ▪ dental pain ▪ dizziness ▪ dyspepsia ▪ fatigue ▪ fever ▪ *headache* ▪ infectious gastroenteritis ▪ influenza ▪ nasal congestion ▪ pyuria ▪ rash ▪ *systemic eosinophilia* ▪ trauma

### Nursing considerations

■ Drug is contraindicated in patients with acute asthmatic attacks or status asthmaticus.

■ Assess patient's underlying condition and monitor patient for effectiveness.
*Alert:* Don't abruptly substitute drug for inhaled or oral corticosteroids. Dosage of inhaled corticosteroids may be reduced gradually.
■ Drug isn't indicated for use in patients with acute asthmatic attacks or status asthmaticus, or as monotherapy for management of exercise-induced bronchospasm. Continue appropriate rescue drug for acute worsening.
■ Give oral granules either directly in the mouth or mixed with a teaspoon of cold or room-temperature applesauce, carrots, rice, or ice cream. Don't open packet until ready to use. After opening packet, give full dose within 15 minutes. If drug is mixed with food, don't store excess for future use; discard any unused portion.
■ Don't dissolve oral granules in liquid; let the patient take a drink after receiving the granules.
■ Oral granules may be given without regard to meals.

# morphine (MOR-feen)

morphine hydrochloride
Morphitec†, M.O.S.†, M.O.S.-S.R.†
morphine sulfate
Astramorph PF, Avinza, Duramorph, Epimorph†, Infumorph, Infumorph 500, Kadian, M-Eslon†, Morphine H.P†, MS Contin, MSIR, MS/L, OMS Concentrate, Oramorph SR, RMS Uniserts, Roxanol, Roxanol 100, Roxanol UD, Statex

Pregnancy risk category: C

## Indications and dosages

### Severe pain

■ *Adults:* 5 to 20 mg subQ or I.M. or 2.5 to 15 mg I.V. q 4 hours, p.r.n. Or, 5 to 30 mg P.O. or 10 to 20 mg P.R. q 4 hours, p.r.n. For continuous I.V. infusion, give loading dose of 15 mg I.V.; then continuous infusion of 0.8 to 10 mg/hour. May also give a 15- or 30-mg extended-release tablet P.O. q 8 to 12 hours. For sustained-release Kadian capsules used as a first opioid, give 20 mg P.O. q 12 hours or 40 mg P.O. once daily; increase conservatively in opioid-naive patients. For epidural injection, give 5 mg by epidural catheter; then, if pain isn't relieved adequately in 1 hour, give supplementary doses of 1 to 2 mg at intervals sufficient to assess efficacy. Maximum epidural dosage, 10 mg/24 hours. For intrathecal injection, a single dose of 0.2 to 1 mg may provide pain relief for 24 hours. Don't repeat injections.
■ *Children:* 0.1 to 0.2 mg/kg subQ or I.M. q 4 hours. Maximum single dose, 15 mg.

### Moderate to severe pain

■ *Adults:* Individualize dosage of Avinza. For patients with no tolerance to opioids, begin with 30 mg Avinza P.O. daily; adjust dosage by no more than 30 mg q 4 days.

## Adverse reactions

Anorexia ■ **apnea** ■ **bradycardia** ■ **cardiac arrest** ■ *clouded sensorium* ■ constipation ■ depression ■ diaphoresis ■ *dizziness* ■ dry mouth ■ edema ■ *euphoria* ■ hallucinations ■ hypertension ■ hypotension ■ ileus ■ *nausea* ■ nervousness ■ *nightmares* ■ physical dependence ■ pruritus and skin flushing ■ **respiratory arrest** ■ **respiratory depression** ■ sedation ■ **seizures** ■ **shock** ■ somnolence ■ syncope ■ tachycardia ■ **thrombocytopenia** ■ urine retention ■ *vomiting*

## Nursing considerations

■ Reassess patient's level of pain at least 15 and 30 minutes after giving parenterally and 30 minutes after giving orally.
■ Keep opioid antagonist and resuscitation equipment available.
**Watch out!** Don't confuse morphine with hydromorphone. Don't confuse Avinza with Invanz.

## naloxone hydrochloride
(nal-OKS-ohn high-droh-KLOR-ighd)

Narcan

Pregnancy risk category: B

### Indications and dosages

**Known or suspected opioid-induced respiratory depression, including that caused by pentazocine and propoxyphene**
■ *Adults:* 0.4 to 2 mg I.V., I.M., or subQ, repeated q 2 to 3 minutes, p.r.n. If there's no response after 10 mg has been given, question diagnosis of opioid-induced toxicity.
■ *Children:* 0.01 mg/kg I.V.; then second dose of 0.1 mg/kg I.V., if needed. If I.V. route isn't available, drug may be given I.M. or subQ in divided doses.
■ *Neonates:* 0.01 mg/kg I.V., I.M., or subQ. Repeat dose q 2 to 3 minutes, p.r.n.

**Postoperative opioid depression**
■ *Adults:* 0.1 to 0.2 mg I.V. q 2 to 3 minutes, p.r.n. Repeat dose within 1 to 2 hours, if needed.
■ *Children:* 0.005 to 0.01 mg I.V. repeated q 2 to 3 minutes, p.r.n.
■ *Neonates (asphyxia neonatorum):* 0.01 mg/kg I.V. into umbilical vein. May be repeated q 2 to 3 minutes.

### Adverse reactions

Diaphoresis ▪ hypertension (with higher-than-recommended doses) ▪ hypotension ▪ nausea ▪ pulmonary edema ▪ *seizures* ▪ tachycardia ▪ tremor ▪ *ventricular fibrillation* ▪ vomiting ▪ withdrawal symptoms in opioid-dependent patients (with higher-than-recommended doses)

### Nursing considerations

■ Naloxone may be given by continous I.V. infusion; usual dosage is 2 mg in 500 ml of $D_5W$ or normal saline solution.
■ Duration of action of the opioid may exceed that of naloxone, and patients may relapse into respiratory depression.
*Alert:* Drug is effective only in reversing respiratory depression caused by opiates.
*Alert:* Monitor respiratory depth and rate. Be prepared to provide oxygen, ventilation, and other resuscitation measures.
**Watch out!** Don't confuse naloxone with naltrexone.

## naltrexone hydrochloride
(nal-TREKS-ohn high-droh-KLOR-ighd)

Depade, ReVia

Pregnancy risk category: C

### Indications and dosages

**Adjunct for maintenance of opioid-free state in detoxified persons**

■ *Adults:* Initially, 25 mg P.O. If no withdrawal signs occur within 1 hour, an additional 25 mg is given. After patient has been started on 50 mg q 24 hours, flexible maintenance schedule may be used. From 50 to 150 mg may be given daily, depending on schedule prescribed.

**Alcohol dependence**

■ *Adults:* 50 mg P.O. once daily.

### Adverse reactions

*Abdominal pain* ● anorexia ● *anxiety* ● chills ● constipation ● decreased potency ● delayed ejaculation ● depression ● dizziness ● fatigue ● *headache* ● **hepatotoxicity** ● increased thirst ● *insomnia* ● *muscle and joint pain* ● nausea ● *nervousness* ● rash ● somnolence ● **suicidal ideation** ● *vomiting*

### Nursing considerations

■ Drug is contraindicated in patients receiving opioid analgesics, in opioid-dependent patients, in patients in acute opioid withdrawal, and in those with positive urine screen for opioids or acute hepatitis or hepatic failure.

■ Treatment for opioid dependence shouldn't begin until patient receives naloxone challenge, a provocative test of opioid dependence. If signs and symptoms of opioid withdrawal persist after naloxone challenge, drug shouldn't be given.

■ Patient must be completely free from opioids before taking drug, or severe withdrawal symptoms may occur. Patients who have been addicted to short-acting opioids, such as heroin and meperidine, must wait at least 7 days after last opioid dose before starting drug. Patients who have been addicted to longer-acting opioids, such as methadone, should wait at least 10 days.

■ In an emergency, anticipate that patient receiving naltrexone may be given an opioid analgesic, but dose must be higher than usual to surmount naltrexone's effect. Watch for respiratory depression from the opioid; it may be longer and deeper.

**Watch out!** Don't confuse naltrexone with naloxone.

## naproxen (nuh-PROK-sin)

naproxen
Apo-Naproxen†, EC-Naprosyn, Naprosyn, Naprosyn-E†, Naprosyn-SR, Naxen†, Novo-Naprox†, Nu-Naprox†
naproxen sodium
Aleve, Anaprox, Anaprox DS, Apo-Napro-Na†, Naprelan, Novo-Naprox Sodium†, Synflex†

Pregnancy risk category: B; D in third trimester

### Indications and dosages

**Rheumatoid arthritis, osteoarthritis, ankylosing spondylitis, pain, dysmenorrhea, tendinitis, bursitis**
■ *Adults:* 250 to 500 mg naproxen b.i.d.; maximum, 1.5 g daily for a limited time. Or, 375 to 500 mg delayed-release EC-Naprosyn b.i.d. Or, 750 to 1,000 mg controlled-release Naprelan daily. Or, 275 to 550 mg naproxen sodium b.i.d.
**Juvenile arthritis**
■ *Children:* 10 mg/kg P.O. in two divided doses.
**Acute gout**
■ *Adults:* 750 mg naproxen P.O.; then 250 mg q 8 hours until attack subsides. Or, 825 mg naproxen sodium; then 275 mg q 8 hours until attack subsides. Or, 1,000 to 1,500 mg daily controlled-release Naprelan on first day; then 1,000 mg daily until attack subsides.
**Mild to moderate pain, primary dysmenorrhea**
■ *Adults:* 500 mg naproxen P.O.; then 250 mg q 6 to 8 hours up to 1.25 g daily. Or, 550 mg naproxen sodium; then 275 mg q 6 to 8 hours up to 1,375 mg daily. Or, 1,000 mg controlled-release Naprelan once daily.
■ *Elderly patients:* For patients older than age 65, don't exceed 400 mg daily.

### Adverse reactions

Abdominal pain • auditory disturbances • constipation • diaphoresis • diarrhea • dizziness • drowsiness • dyspepsia • dyspnea • ecchymoses • edema • epigastric pain • headache • heartburn • **hyperkalemia** • increased bleeding time • nausea • occult blood loss • palpitations • peptic ulceration • pruritus • purpura • rash • stomatitis • thirst • *tinnitus* • urticaria • vertigo • vision disturbances

### Nursing considerations

■ Drug is contraindicated in patients with asthma, rhinitis, or nasal polyps.
■ Because NSAIDs impair synthesis of renal prostaglandins, they can decrease renal blood flow and lead to reversible renal impairment, especially in patients with renal failure, heart failure, or hepatic dysfunction; in elderly patients; and in those taking diuretics. NSAIDs may mask signs and symptoms of infection.

# nesiritide (neh-SIR-ih-tide)

Natrecor

*Pregnancy risk category: C*

## Indications and dosages

**Acutely decompensated heart failure in patients with dyspnea at rest or with minimal activity**

■ *Adults:* 2 mcg/kg by I.V. bolus over 60 seconds, followed by continuous infusion of 0.01 mcg/kg/minute.

*Adjust-a-dose:* If hypotension develops during administration, reduce dosage or stop drug. Restart drug at dosage reduced by 30% with no bolus doses.

## Adverse reactions

Abdominal pain ● anemia ● angina ● anxiety ● **apnea** ● atrial fibrillation ● AV node conduction abnormalities ● back pain ● ***bradycardia*** ● confusion ● cough ● diaphoresis ● dizziness ● fever ● headache ● *hypotension* ● injection site reactions ● insomnia ● leg cramps ● nausea ● pain at injection site ● paresthesia ● pruritus ● rash ● somnolence ● tremor ● ventricular extrasystoles ● ***ventricular tachycardia*** ● vomiting

## Nursing considerations

■ Drug is contraindicated in patients with cardiogenic shock, systolic blood pressure below 90 mm Hg, low cardiac filling pressures, conditions in which cardiac output depends on venous return, or conditions that make vasodilators inappropriate, such as valvular stenosis, restrictive or obstructive cardiomyopathy, constrictive pericarditis, and pericardial tamponade.

■ Reconstitute one 1.5-mg vial with 5 ml of diluent (such as $D_5W$) from a prefilled 250-ml I.V. bag. Gently rock vial until solution becomes clear and colorless; withdraw contents of vial and add back to the 250-ml I.V. bag to yield 6 mcg/ml. Invert the bag several times to ensure complete mixing, and use the solution within 24 hours.

■ Use the formulas below to calculate bolus volume (2 mcg/kg) and infusion flow rate (0.01 mcg/kg/minute):

Bolus volume (ml) =
0.33 × patient weight (kg)

Infusion flow rate (ml/hr) =
0.1 × patient weight (kg)

■ Before giving bolus dose, prime I.V. tubing. Withdraw bolus and give over 60 seconds through an I.V. port in tubing.

■ Immediately after giving bolus, infuse drug at 0.1 ml/kg/hour to deliver 0.01 mcg/kg/minute.

■ Monitor patient's blood pressure closely, particularly if he's also taking an ACE inhibitor.

# nifedipine (nigh-FEH-duh-peen)

Adalat, Adalat CC, Adalat P.A.†, Adalat XL†, Apo-Nifed†, Nifedical XL, Novo-Nifedin†, Nu-Nifed†, Procardia XL

Pregnancy risk category: C

## Indications and dosages

**Vasospastic angina (Prinzmetal's or variant angina), classic chronic stable angina pectoris**

■ *Adults:* Initially, 10 mg (short-acting capsules) P.O. t.i.d. Usual effective dosage, 10 to 20 mg t.i.d. Some patients may require up to 30 mg q.i.d. Maximum dosage, 180 mg daily. Adjust dosage over 7 to 14 days to evaluate response. Or, 30 to 60 mg (extended-release tablets, except Adalat CC) P.O. once daily. Maximum dosage, 120 mg daily. Adjust dosage over 7 to 14 days to evaluate response.

**Hypertension**

■ *Adults:* 30 or 60 mg P.O. (extended-release) once daily; adjust over 7 to 14 days. Doses larger than 90 mg (Adalat CC) and 120 mg (Procardia XL) aren't recommended.

## Adverse reactions

Abdominal discomfort ▪ constipation ▪ cough ▪ diarrhea ▪ *dizziness* ▪ dyspnea ▪ *flushing* ▪ *headache* ▪ **heart failure** ▪ hypotension ▪ *lightheadedness* ▪ *MI* ▪ muscle cramps ▪ nasal congestion ▪ *nausea* ▪ nervousness ▪ palpitations ▪ *peripheral edema* ▪ pruritus ▪ pulmonary edema ▪ rash ▪ somnolence ▪ syncope ▪ *weakness*

## Nursing considerations

■ Don't give immediate-release form within 1 week of acute MI or in acute coronary syndrome.

■ Monitor blood pressure regularly, especially in patients who take beta-adrenergic blockers or antihypertensives.

■ Watch for symptoms of heart failure.

■ Although rebound effect hasn't been observed when drug is stopped, reduce dosage slowly under prescriber's supervision.

**Watch out!** Don't confuse nifedipine with nicardipine or nimodipine.

# nitroglycerin (nigh-troh-GLIH-suh-rin)

Deponit, Minitran, Nitrek, Nitro-Bid, Nitro-Bid IV, Nitrodisc, Nitro-Dur, Nitrogard, Nitroglyn, Nitrolingual, Nitrong, NitroQuick, Nitrostat, NitroTab, Nitro-Time, Transderm-Nitro, Tridil

*Pregnancy risk category: C*

## Indications and dosages

**Prophylaxis against chronic anginal attacks**
■ *Adults:* 2.5 or 2.6 mg sustained-release capsule or tablet q 8 to 12 hours, adjusted upward to an effective dose in 2.5- or 2.6-mg increments b.i.d. to q.i.d. Or, use 2% ointment: Start with ½-inch ointment, increasing by ½-inch increments until desired results are achieved. Ointment dosage range, ½ to 5 inches. Usual dosage, 1 to 2 inches q 6 to 8 hours. Or, transdermal disc or pad (Nitrodisc, Nitro-Dur, or Transderm-Nitro) 0.2 to 0.4 mg/hour once daily.

**Acute angina pectoris, prophylaxis to prevent or minimize anginal attacks before stressful events**
■ *Adults:* 1 S.L. tablet (1/400 grain, 1/200 grain, 1/150 grain, 1/100 grain) dissolved under the tongue or in the buccal pouch as soon as angina begins; repeat q 5 minutes, if needed, for 15 minutes. Or, one or two sprays (Nitrolingual) into mouth, preferably onto or under the tongue; repeat q 3 to 5 minutes, if needed, to maximum of three doses within a 15-minute period. Or, 1 to 3 mg transmucosally q 3 to 5 hours while awake.

**Hypertension from surgery, heart failure after MI, angina pectoris in acute situations, to produce controlled hypotension during surgery (by I.V. infusion)**
■ *Adults:* Initially, infuse at 5 mcg/minute, increasing, p.r.n., by 5 mcg/minute q 3 to 5 minutes until response occurs. If a 20-mcg/minute rate doesn't produce a response, increase dosage by as much as 20 mcg/minute q 3 to 5 minutes. Up to 100 mcg/minute may be needed.

## Adverse reactions

Contact dermatitis ● cutaneous vasodilation ● *dizziness* ● fainting ● *flushing* ● *headache* ● hypersensitivity reaction ● nausea ● *orthostatic hypotension* ● *palpitations* ● rash ● S.L. burning ● *tachycardia* ● vomiting ● weakness

## Nursing considerations

■ Drug is contraindicated in patients with early MI (P.O. and S.L.), severe anemia, increased intracranial pressure, angle-closure glaucoma, orthostatic hypotension, allergy to adhesives (transdermal), or hypersensitivity to nitrates. I.V. nitroglycerin is contraindicated in patients hypersensitive to I.V. form and in those with cardiac tamponade, restrictive cardiomyopathy, or constrictive pericarditis.

## nitroglycerin *(continued)*

■ Dilute I.V. form with D$_5$W or normal saline solution for injection. Concentration shouldn't exceed 400 mcg/ml.
■ Always give I.V. form with an infusion control device and titrate to desired response.
■ Always mix in glass bottles, and avoid use of I.V. filters because drug binds to plastic. Regular polyvinyl chloride tubing can bind up to 80% of drug, making it necessary to infuse higher dosages.
■ When changing the concentration of infusion, flush the I.V. administration set with 15 to 20 ml of the new concentration before use. This will clear the line of old drug solution.
■ Closely monitor vital signs, particularly blood pressure, during infusion, especially in a patient with MI. Excessive hypotension may worsen MI.
■ To apply ointment, measure prescribed amount on application paper; then place paper on any nonhairy area. Don't rub in. Cover with plastic film to aid absorption and protect clothing. Remove all excess ointment from previous site before applying next dose. Avoid getting ointment on fingers.
■ Transdermal dosage forms can be applied to any nonhairy part of skin except distal parts of arms and legs (absorption won't be maximal at distal sites). Patch may cause contact dermatitis.

■ Remove transdermal patch before defibrillation. Because of the aluminum backing on patch, the electric current may cause arcing that can damage the paddles and burn the patient.
■ When stopping transdermal treatment of angina, expect to gradually reduce dosage and frequency of application over 4 to 6 weeks.
■ Monitor blood pressure and intensity and duration of drug response.
■ Drug may cause headaches, especially at beginning of therapy. Dosage may be reduced temporarily, but tolerance usually develops. Treat headache with aspirin or acetaminophen.
■ Tolerance to drug can be minimized with a 10- to 12-hour nitrate-free interval. To achieve this, remove the transdermal system in the early evening and apply a new system the next morning, or omit the last daily dose of a buccal, sustained-release, or ointment form. Check with the prescriber for alterations in dosage regimen if tolerance is suspected.
**Watch out!** Don't confuse nitroglycerin with nitroprusside. Don't confuse Nitro-Bid with Nicobid.

# nitroprusside sodium
(nigh-troh-PRUS-ighd SOH-dee-um)

Nipride†, Nitropress

Pregnancy risk category: C

## Indications and dosages

**To lower blood pressure quickly in hypertensive emergencies, to produce controlled hypotension during anesthesia, to reduce preload and afterload in cardiac pump failure or cardiogenic shock (used with or without dopamine)**
■ *Adults and children:* Begin infusion at 0.25 to 0.3 mcg/kg/minute I.V. and gradually titrate q few minutes to maximum infusion rate of 10 mcg/kg/minute.
*Adjust-a-dose:* Patients taking other antihypertensives with nitroprusside are extremely sensitive to nitroprusside. Titrate dosage accordingly. Use with caution in patients with renal failure; reduce dosage as much as possible.

## Adverse reactions

*Abdominal pain* ▪ acidosis ▪ apprehension ▪ **bradycardia** ▪ **cyanide toxicity** ▪ *diaphoresis* ▪ *dizziness* ▪ ECG changes ▪ flushing ▪ *headache* ▪ hypotension ▪ hypothyroidism ▪ ileus ▪ **increased intracranial pressure** ▪ irritation at infusion site ▪ loss of consciousness ▪ **methemoglobinemia** ▪ *muscle twitching* ▪ *nausea* ▪ palpitations ▪ pink color ▪ rash ▪ restlessness ▪ tachycardia ▪ **thiocyante toxicity** ▪ venous streaking

## Nursing considerations

■ Drug is contraindicated in patients with compensatory hypertension (such as in arteriovenous shunt or coarctation of the aorta), inadequate cerebral circulation, acute heart failure with reduced peripheral vascular resistance, congenital optic atrophy, or tobacco-induced amblyopia.
*Alert:* Excessive doses or infusing at a rate greater than 10 mcg/kg/minute can cause cyanide toxicity. Check thiocyanate level every 72 hours; a level higher than 100 mcg/ml may be toxic.
■ Because drug is sensitive to light, wrap I.V. solution in foil or other opaque material; it isn't necessary to wrap tubing. Fresh solution should have faint brownish tint.
■ Infuse with an infusion pump.
■ Check blood pressure every 5 minutes at start of infusion and every 15 minutes thereafter.
■ If severe hypotension occurs, stop nitroprusside infusion; effects of drug quickly reverse.
**Watch out!** Don't confuse nitroprusside with nitroglycerin.

# norepinephrine bitartrate
(nor-ep-ih-NEF-rin bigh-TAR-trayt)

Levophed

Pregnancy risk category: C

## Indications and dosages

**To restore blood pressure in acute hypotensive states**

■ *Adults:* Initially, 8 to 12 mcg/minute by I.V. infusion; then titrate to maintain normal blood pressure. Average maintenance dosage, 2 to 4 mcg/minute.

■ *Children:* 2 mcg/minute or 2 mcg/m$^2$/minute by I.V. infusion; adjust dosage based on response.

**Severe hypotension during cardiac arrest**

■ *Children:* Initially, 0.1 mcg/kg/minute I.V. infusion. Titrate infusion rate based on response up to 2 mcg/kg/minute.

## Adverse reactions

**Anaphylaxis** • anxiety • **arrhythmias** • **asthma attacks** • **bradycardia** • dizziness • *headache* • insomnia • irritation with extravasation • necrosis and gangrene secondary to extravasation • respiratory difficulties • restlessness • *severe hypertension* • tremor • weakness

## Nursing considerations

■ Drug is contraindicated in patients with mesenteric or peripheral vascular thrombosis, profound hypoxia, hypercarbia, or hypotension resulting from blood volume deficit.

■ Drug is contraindicated during cyclopropane and halothane anesthesia.

■ Use a central venous catheter or large vein, as in the antecubital fossa, to minimize risk of extravasation. Give in $D_5W$ or normal saline solution for injection. Use continuous infusion pump to regulate flow rate and a piggyback setup so I.V. line stays open if norepinephrine is stopped.

■ Check site frequently for signs of extravasation. If they appear, stop infusion immediately and notify prescriber. Infiltrate area with 5 to 10 mg phentolamine in 10 to 15 ml of normal saline solution to counteract effect of extravasation.

■ Protect drug from light. Discard discolored solutions or solutions that contain a precipitate. Norepinephrine solutions deteriorate after 24 hours.

*Alert:* Never leave patient unattended during infusion. Check blood pressure every 2 minutes until stabilized; then check every 5 minutes.

■ Frequently monitor ECG, cardiac output, central venous pressure, pulmonary artery wedge pressure, pulse rate, urine output, and color and temperature of limbs.

**Watch out!** Don't confuse norepinephrine with epinephrine.

# nystatin (nigh-STAT-in)

Mycostatin, Nilstat, Nystex, Pedi-Dri

Pregnancy risk category: NR

## Indications and dosages

**Cutaneous and mucocutaneous infections caused by *Candida albicans***

■ *Adults and children:* Apply to affected area up to several times daily until healing is complete. Apply cream or ointment b.i.d. or as indicated; powder, b.i.d. or t.i.d.; lozenges, 1 or 2 four to five times daily until 48 hours after oral symptoms subside, but not longer than 14 days; suspension, 4 to 6 ml q.i.d. (one-half of dose in each side of mouth); retain dose as long as possible before swallowing.

**Vulvovaginal candidiasis**

■ *Adults:* 1 vaginal tablet daily for 14 days.

## Adverse reactions

Occasional contact dermatitis from preservatives in some forms

## Nursing considerations

■ Don't use occlusive dressings.
■ Preparation doesn't stain skin or mucous membranes.
■ Cream is recommended for skinfolds; powder, for moist areas; ointment, for dry areas.
**Watch out!** Don't confuse nystatin with Nitrostat.

## olanzapine (oh-LAN-za-peen)

Zyprexa, Zyprexa Zydis

Pregnancy risk category: C

### Indications and dosages

**Schizophrenia**

■ *Adults:* Initially, 5 to 10 mg P.O. once daily with goal of 10 mg daily. Adjust dosage in 5-mg increments at intervals of 1 week or more.

**Short-term treatment of acute manic episodes linked to bipolar I disorder**

■ *Adults:* Initially, 10 to 15 mg P.O. daily. Adjust dosage, p.r.n., in 5-mg daily increments at intervals of 24 hours or more. Maximum, 20 mg P.O. daily. Duration of treatment is 3 to 4 weeks.

**Short-term treatment of acute manic episodes linked to bipolar I disorder**

■ *Adults:* 10 mg P.O. once daily. Dosage range, 5 to 20 mg daily. Duration of treatment is 6 weeks.

**Long-term treatment of bipolar I disorder**

■ *Adults:* 5 to 20 mg P.O. daily.

**Adjunct to lithium or valproate to treat bipolar mania**

■ *Adults:* 10 mg P.O. daily. Usual range, 5 to 20 mg daily.

*Adjust-a-dose:* For elderly or debilitated patients, those predisposed to hypotension, and those who may be sensitive to olanzapine, initially, 5 mg P.O. daily. Increase dosage cautiously.

**Agitation caused by schizophrenia and bipolar I mania**

■ *Adults:* 10 mg I.M. Subsequent doses of up to 10 mg may be given 2 hours after first dose or 4 hours after second dose, up to 30 mg I.M. daily. Maintenance dose, 5 to 20 mg P.O. daily.

*Adjust-a-dose:* For elderly patients, give 5 mg I.M. For debilitated patients, those predisposed to hypotension, and patients sensitive to effects of olanzapine, give 2.5 mg I.M.

### Adverse reactions

Amblyopia ▪ amenorrhea ▪ back pain ▪ chest pain ▪ *constipation* ▪ dizziness ▪ dry mouth ▪ dyspepsia ▪ dyspnea ▪ extrapyramidal events ▪ fever ▪ flulike syndrome ▪ hematuria ▪ *hyperglycemia* ▪ hypertension ▪ hypotension (with I.M. route) ▪ increased appetite ▪ cough ▪ *insomnia* ▪ joint pain ▪ **leukopenia** ▪ **neuroleptic malignant syndrome** ▪ orthostatic hypotension ▪ *parkinsonism* ▪ edema ▪ pharyngitis ▪ rhinitis ▪ *somnolence* ▪ **suicide attempt** ▪ sweating ▪ tachycardia ▪ UTI ▪ vomiting

### Nursing considerations

■ Monitor patient for abnormal body temperature regulation.
■ Obtain baseline and periodic liver function test results.
**Watch out!** Don't confuse olanzapine with olsalazine. Don't confuse Zyprexa with Zyrtec.

O-R

# omeprazole (oh-MEH-pruh-zohl)

omeprazole
Losec†, Prilosec, Zegerid‡
omeprazole magnesium
Prilosec OTC

Pregnancy risk category: C

## Indications and dosages

**Symptomatic gastroesophageal reflux disease (GERD) without esophageal lesions**
■ *Adults:* 20 mg P.O. as delayed-release or oral suspension, daily for 4 weeks for patients who respond poorly to H$_2$-receptor antagonists.

**Erosive esophagitis and accompanying symptoms of GERD**
■ *Adults:* 20 mg P.O. daily for 4 to 8 weeks.

**Maintenance of healing erosive esophagitis**
■ *Adults:* 20 mg P.O. as delayed-release or oral suspension, daily.

**Pathologic hypersecretory conditions**
■ *Adults:* Initially, 60 mg P.O. daily; adjust dosage. If daily dose exceeds 80 mg, give in divided doses. Doses up to 120 mg t.i.d. have been given. Continue therapy p.r.n.

**Duodenal ulcer**
■ *Adults:* 20 mg P.O. as delayed-release or oral suspension, daily for 4 to 8 weeks.

**Helicobacter pylori infection and duodenal ulcer disease**
■ *Adults:* 40 mg P.O. q morning with clarithromycin 500 mg P.O. t.i.d. for 14 days. For patients with an ulcer at start of therapy,

*160*

give another 14 days of omeprazole 20 mg P.O. once daily.

**H. pylori infection and duodenal ulcer disease (with clarithromycin and amoxicillin)**
■ *Adults:* 20 mg P.O. with clarithromycin 500 mg P.O. and amoxicillin 1,000 mg P.O., each given b.i.d. for 10 days. For patients with ulcers at start of therapy, give another 18 days of omeprazole 20 mg P.O. once daily.

**Short-term treatment of active benign gastric ulcer**
■ *Adults:* 40 mg P.O. once daily for 4 to 8 weeks.

**Frequent heartburn**
■ *Adults:* 20 mg P.O. Prilosec OTC once daily before breakfast for 14 days. May repeat course q 4 months.

## Adverse reactions

Abdominal pain • asthenia • back pain • constipation • cough • diarrhea • dizziness • flatulence • headache • nausea • rash • vomiting

## Nursing considerations

■ Zegerid is contraindicated in patients with metabolic alkalosis or hypocalcemia.

**Watch out!** Don't confuse Prilosec with Prilocaine, Prinivil, or Prozac.

# oxytocin, synthetic injection
(oks-ih-TOH-sin, sin-THET-ik in-JEK-shun)

Pitocin

Pregnancy risk category: NR

## Indications and dosages

**To induce or stimulate labor**

■ *Adults:* Initially, 10 units in 1,000 ml of $D_5W$, lactated Ringer's, or normal saline solution I.V. infused at 1 to 2 milliunits/minute. Increase rate by 1 to 2 milliunits/minute at 15- to 30-minute intervals until normal contraction pattern is established. Decrease rate when labor is firmly established. Maximum dosage, 20 milliunits/minute.

**To reduce postpartum bleeding after expulsion of placenta**

■ *Adults:* 10 to 40 units in 1,000 ml of $D_5W$, lactated Ringer's, or normal saline solution I.V. infused at rate needed to control bleeding, usually 20 to 40 milliunits/minute. 10 units may be given I.M. after delivery of placenta.

**Incomplete or inevitable abortion**

■ *Adults:* 10 units I.V. in 500 ml of normal saline, lactated Ringer's, or dextrose 5% in normal saline solution. Infuse at 10 to 20 milliunits/minute.

## Adverse reactions

### Maternal

*Abruptio placentae* • *afibrinogenemia* • *arrhythmias* • *anaphylaxis* • *coma* • *death* • hypersensitivity reactions • hypertension • impaired uterine blood flow • increased heart rate, *postpartum hemorrhage* • increased uterine motility • nausea • pelvic hematoma • *seizures* • *subarachnoid hemorrhage* • tetanic uterine contractions • *uterine rupture* • vomiting

### Fetal

*Anoxia* • *asphyxia* • *arrhythmias* • *bradycardia* • *brain damage* • *low Apgar scores at 5 minutes* • neonatal jaundice • neonatal retinal hemorrhage

## Nursing considerations

■ Drug is contraindicated when vaginal delivery isn't advised (placenta previa, vasa previa, invasive cervical carcinoma, genital herpes), with cephalopelvic disproportion, or when delivery requires conversion.

■ Drug is contraindicated in fetal distress when delivery isn't imminent, in prematurity, in other obstetric emergencies, and in patients with severe toxemia or hypertonic uterine patterns.

■ Have 20% magnesium sulfate solution available to relax the myometrium.

■ If contractions occur less than 2 minutes apart, exceed 50 mm, or last 90 seconds or longer, stop infusion, turn patient on her side, and notify prescriber.

**Watch out!** Don't confuse Pitocin with Pitressin.

# pantoprazole sodium (pan-TOE-prah-zole)

Protonix, Protonix IV

*Pregnancy risk category:* **B**

## Indications and dosages

*Note:* Stop treatment with I.V. form when P.O. form is warranted.

**Erosive esophagitis with gastro-esophageal reflux disease (GERD)**
■ *Adults:* 40 mg P.O. once daily for up to 8 weeks. For patients who haven't healed after 8 weeks of treatment, another 8-week course may be considered.

**Short-term treatment of GERD in patients who can't take delayed-release tablets orally**
■ *Adults:* 40 mg I.V. daily for 7 to 10 days.

**Short-term treatment of GERD linked to history of erosive esophagitis**
■ *Adults:* 40 mg I.V. once daily for 7 to 10 days. Switch to P.O. form as soon as patient is able.

**Long-term maintenance of healing erosive esophagitis and reduction in relapse rates of daytime and nighttime heartburn symptoms in patients with GERD**
■ *Adults:* 40 mg P.O. once daily.

**Short-term treatment of patho-logic hypersecretion conditions**
■ *Adults:* Individualize dosage. Usual dosage is 80 mg I.V. q 12 hours for no more than 6 days. Dosage of 80 mg q 8 hours may be required. Maximum dosage, 240 mg/day.

**Long-term treatment of patho-logic hypersecretory conditions**
■ *Adults:* Individualize dosage. Usual starting dosage is 40 mg P.O. b.i.d. Adjust dosage to a maximum of 240 mg/day.

## Adverse reactions

Abdominal pain ▪ anxiety ▪ arthral-gia ▪ asthenia ▪ back pain ▪ bron-chitis ▪ chest pain ▪ constipation ▪ diarrhea ▪ dizziness ▪ dyspepsia ▪ dyspnea ▪ eructation ▪ flatulence ▪ flulike syndrome ▪ gastroenter-itis ▪ headache ▪ hyperglycemia ▪ hyperlipemia ▪ hypertonia ▪ in-creased cough ▪ infection ▪ in-somnia ▪ migraine ▪ nausea ▪ neck pain ▪ pharyngitis ▪ rash ▪ sinusi-tis ▪ upper respiratory tract infec-tion ▪ urinary frequency ▪ UTI ▪ vomiting

## Nursing considerations

■ Infuse diluted solutions I.V. over 15 minutes at a rate of about 7 ml/minute.

**Watch out!** Don't confuse Protonix with Prevacid, Prilosec, or Prozac

# paroxetine hydrochloride
(par-OKS-eh-teen high-droh-KLOR-ighd)

Paxil, Paxil CR

Pregnancy risk category: C

## Indications and dosages

### Depression

■ *Adults:* Initially, 20 mg P.O. daily. May increase dosage by 10 mg daily at 1 week intervals to maximum of 50 mg daily. Controlled-release form, initially 25 mg P.O. daily. May increase dosage by 12.5 mg daily at weekly intervals, up to 62.5 mg daily.

### Obsessive-compulsive disorder

■ *Adults:* Initially, 20 mg P.O. daily. May increase dosage by 10 mg daily at weekly intervals. Recommended dosage, 40 mg daily.

### Panic disorder

■ *Adults:* Initially, 10 mg P.O. daily. May increase dosage by 10 mg at weekly intervals, to maximum of 60 mg daily. Or, 12.5 mg (Paxil CR) P.O. as a single daily dose. May increase dosage at weekly intervals by 12.5 mg daily, up to 75 mg daily.
*Adjust-a-dose:* For elderly or debilitated patients and those with severe renal or hepatic impairment, first dose of Paxil CR should be 12.5 mg daily; may increase if indicated. Don't exceed 50 mg daily.

### Social anxiety disorder

■ *Adults:* Initially, 20 mg P.O. daily. Dosage range, 20 to 60 mg daily. Or, 12.5 mg (Paxil CR) P.O. as a single daily dose. Increase dosage at weekly intervals in increments of 12.5 mg daily, Don't exceed 37.5 mg daily.

### Generalized anxiety disorder

■ *Adults:* Initially, 20 mg P.O. daily, increasing by 10 mg/day weekly up to 50 mg daily.
*Adjust-a-dose:* For debilitated patients and those with renal or hepatic impairment who are taking immediate-release form, initially 10 mg P.O. daily. May increase dosage by 10 mg/day at weekly intervals, to maximum of 40 mg daily. If using Paxil CR, initially 12.5 mg daily, not to exceed 50 mg daily.

## Adverse reactions

Agitation ▪ anxiety ▪ *asthenia* ▪ confusion ▪ *constipation* ▪ *diaphoresis* ▪ *diarrhea* ▪ *dizziness* ▪ *dry mouth* ▪ flatulence ▪ *headache* ▪ appetite changes ▪ *insomnia* ▪ myalgia ▪ myasthenia ▪ *nausea* ▪ *nervousness* ▪ orthostatic hypotension ▪ palpitations ▪ paresthesia ▪ pruritus ▪ rash ▪ *sexual dysfunction* ▪ *somnolence* ▪ **suicidal behavior** ▪ tremor ▪ urinary frequency ▪ vomiting

## Nursing considerations

■ Drug is contraindicated within 14 days of MAO inhibitor therapy and in those taking thioridazine.
■ Monitor patient for suicidal tendencies.
**Watch out!** Don't confuse paroxetine with paclitaxel. Don't confuse Paxil with Doxil, paclitaxel, Plavix, or Taxol.

O-R

# penicillin V potassium
## (pen-ih-SIL-in VEE poh-TAS-ee-um)

Apo-Pen-VK†, Nadopen-V 200†, Nadopen-V 400†, Novo-Pen-VK†, Nu-Pen-VK†, Pen Vee†, PVF K†, Veetids

Pregnancy risk category: B

## Indications and dosages

### Mild to moderate systemic infections

■ *Adults and children age 12 and older:* 125 to 500 mg P.O. q 6 hours.
■ *Children younger than age 12:* 15 to 62.5 mg/kg P.O. daily in divided doses q 6 to 8 hours.

### To prevent recurrent rheumatic fever

■ *Adults and children:* 250 mg P.O. b.i.d.

## Off-label uses

### Erythema chronica migrans in Lyme disease

■ *Adults:* 250 to 500 mg P.O. q.i.d. for 10 to 20 days.
■ *Children younger than age 2:* 50 mg/kg/day (up to 2 g/day) P.O. in four divided doses for 10 to 20 days.

### To prevent inhalation anthrax after possible exposure

■ *Adults:* 7.5 mg/kg P.O. q.i.d. Continue treatment until exposure is ruled out. If exposure is confirmed, anthrax vaccine may be indicated. Continue treatment for 60 days.
■ *Children younger than age 9:* 50 mg/kg P.O. daily given in four divided doses. Continue treatment until exposure is ruled out. If exposure is confirmed, anthrax vaccine may be indicated. Continue treatment for 60 days.

## Adverse reactions

**Anaphylaxis** ● black hairy tongue ● diarrhea ● eosinophilia ● *epigastric distress* ● hemolytic anemia ● hypersensitivity reactions ● **leukopenia** ● *nausea* ● nephropathy ● neuropathy ● overgrowth of non-susceptible organisms ● **thrombocytopenia** ● vomiting

## Nursing considerations

■ Before giving drug, ask patient about allergic reactions to penicillins.
■ Obtain specimen for culture and sensitivity testing before giving first dose. Therapy may begin pending results.
■ Periodically assess renal and hematopoietic function in patients receiving long-term therapy.
■ Watch for signs and symptoms of superinfection.
■ The American Heart Association considers amoxicillin the preferred drug to prevent endocarditis; however, penicillin V is considered an alternative drug.
**Watch out!** Don't confuse penicillin V potassium with penicillamine, Polycillin, or the various types of penicillin.

## pentoxifylline (pen-tok-SIH-fi-lin)

Trental

Pregnancy risk category: C

### Indications and dosages

**Intermittent claudication from chronic occlusive vascular disease**
■ *Adults:* 400 mg P.O. t.i.d. with meals. May decrease to 400 mg b.i.d. if GI and CNS adverse effects occur.

### Adverse reactions

Dizziness • dyspepsia • headache • nausea • vomiting

### Nursing considerations

▢ Drug is contraindicated in patients intolerant to methylxanthines, such as caffeine, theophyl-line, and theo-bromine, and in those with recent cerebral or retinal hemorrhage.
▢ Drug is useful in patients who aren't good surgical candidates.
▢ Elderly patients may be more sensitive to drug's effects.
**Watch out!** Don't confuse Trental with Trandate.

# phenylephrine hydrochloride
(fen-il-EF-rin high-droh-KLOR-ighd)

Neo-Synephrine

Pregnancy risk category: C

## Indications and dosages

**Hypotensive emergencies during spinal anesthesia**
■ *Adults:* Initially, 0.2 mg I.V.; don't let subsequent doses exceed the preceding dose by more than 0.2 mg. Maximum single dose, 0.5 mg.

**To maintain blood pressure during spinal or inhaled anesthesia**
■ *Adults:* 2 to 3 mg subQ or I.M. 3 to 4 minutes before anesthesia.
■ *Children:* 0.044 to 0.088 mg/kg subQ or I.M.

**To prolong spinal anesthesia**
■ *Adults:* 2 to 5 mg added to anesthetic solution.

**Vasoconstrictor for regional anesthesia**
■ *Adults:* 1 mg phenylephrine per 20 ml of local anesthetic.

**Mild to moderate hypotension**
■ *Adults:* 2 to 5 mg subQ or I.M.; repeat in 1 or 2 hours p.r.n. and as tolerated. First dose shouldn't exceed 5 mg. Or, 0.1 to 0.5 mg slow I.V., not to be repeated more often than q 10 to 15 minutes.
■ *Children:* 0.1 mg/kg or 3 mg/m² I.M. or subQ; repeat in 1 or 2 hours as needed and tolerated.

**Severe hypotension and shock**
■ *Adults:* 10 mg in 250 to 500 ml of $D_5W$ or normal saline solution for injection. Start I.V. infusion at 100 to 180 mcg/minute; then de-

crease to maintenance infusion of 40 to 60 mcg/minute when blood pressure stabilizes.

**Paroxysmal supraventricular tachycardia**
■ *Adults:* Initially, 0.5 mg by rapid I.V. injection; increase in increments of 0.1 to 0.2 mg. Use cautiously. Maximum single dose, 1 mg.

## Adverse reactions

*Anaphylaxis* • anxiety • *arrhythmias* • *asthmatic episodes* • dizziness • excitability • headache • hypertension • restlessness • tachyphylaxis and decreased organ perfusion • tissue sloughing (with extravasation) • weakness

## Nursing considerations

■ Drug is contraindicated in patients with severe hypertension or ventricular tachycardia.
■ To treat extravasation, infiltrate site promptly with 10 to 15 ml of normal saline solution for injection containing 5 to 10 mg phentolamine. Use a fine needle.
■ During infusion, frequently monitor ECG, blood pressure, cardiac output, central venous pressure, pulmonary artery wedge pressure, pulse rate, urine output, and color and temperature of limbs.

## phenytoin (FEN-uh-toyn)

phenytoin
**Dilantin-125, Dilantin Infatabs**
phenytoin sodium (prompt)
**Dilantin**
phenytoin sodium (extended)
**Dilantin Kapseals, Phenytek**

Pregnancy risk category: **D**

### Indications and dosages

**To control tonic-clonic (grand mal) and complex partial (temporal lobe) seizures**

■ *Adults:* Highly individualized. Initially, 100 mg P.O. t.i.d., increasing by 100 mg P.O. q 2 to 4 weeks until desired response. Usual dosage range, 300 to 600 mg daily. If patient is stabilized, once-daily dosing with 300-mg extended-release capsules is a possible alternative.

■ *Children:* 5 mg/kg or 250 mg/m$^2$ P.O. divided b.i.d. or t.i.d. Usual dosage range, 4 to 8 mg/kg daily. Maximum dosage, 300 mg daily.

**For patient requiring a loading dose**

■ *Adults:* Initially, 1 g P.O. daily divided into three doses and given at 2-hour intervals. Or, 10 to 15 mg/kg I.V. at a rate not exceeding 50 mg/minute. Normal maintenance dosage is started 24 hours after loading dose.

■ *Children:* 500 to 600 mg P.O. in divided doses, followed by maintenance dosage 24 hours after loading dose.

**To prevent and treat seizures occurring during neurosurgery**

■ *Adults:* 100 to 200 mg I.M. q 4 hours during and after surgery.

**Status epilepticus**

■ *Adults:* Loading dose of 10 to 15 mg/kg I.V. (1 to 1.5 g may be needed) at a rate not exceeding 50 mg/minute; then maintenance dosage of 100 mg P.O. or I.V. q 6 to 8 hours.

■ *Children:* Loading dose of 15 to 20 mg/kg I.V. at a rate not exceeding 3 mg/kg/minute; then highly individualized maintenance dosages.

*Adjust-a-dose:* Elderly patients may need lower dosages.

### Adverse reactions

**Agranulocytosis** • ataxia • blurred vision • bullous or purpuric dermatitis • constipation • *decreased coordination* • *diplopia* • discoloration of skin (if given by I.V. push in back of hand) • dizziness • exfoliative dermatitis • *gingival hyperplasia* • headache • *hirsutism* • hyperglycemia • hypertrichosis • inflammation and necrosis at injection site • insomnia • **leukopenia** • lupus erythematosus • lymphadenopathy • macrocy-

*(continued)*

## phenytoin (continued)

themia • megaloblastic anemia • *mental confusion* • nausea • nervousness • *nystagmus* • osteomalacia • pain • **pancytopenia** • periarteritis nodosa • photosensitivity reaction • scarlatiniform or morbilliform rash • *slurred speech* • **Stevens-Johnson syndrome** • **thrombocytopenia** • **toxic epidermal necrolysis** • **toxic hepatitis** • twitching • *vomiting*

### Nursing considerations

• Drug is contraindicated in patients with sinus bradycardia, sinoatrial block, second- or third-degree atrioventricular block, or Adams-Stokes syndrome.

• Give I.V. bolus slowly (50 mg/minute).

• If giving as an infusion, don't mix drug with $D_5W$ because it will precipitate.

• Clear I.V. tubing first with normal saline solution. Never use cloudy solution.

• Mix with normal saline solution, if needed, and give as an infusion over 30 minutes to 1 hour, when possible. Infusion must begin within 1 hour after preparation and should run through an inline filter.

*Alert:* Check patency of I.V. catheter before giving. Monitor I.V. site for extravasation because it can cause severe tissue damage.

• If possible, don't give phenytoin by I.V. push into veins on back of hand to avoid discoloration (purple-glove syndrome). Inject into larger veins or central venous catheter, if available.

• Check vital signs, blood pressure, and ECG during I.V. administration.

• Phenytoin requirements usually increase during pregnancy.

• Use only clear solution for injection. A slight yellow color is acceptable. Don't refrigerate.

• Don't give I.M. unless dosage adjustments are made; drug may precipitate at injection site, cause pain, and be absorbed erratically.

• Divided doses given with or after meals may decrease adverse GI reactions.

• Stop drug if rash appears.

• Don't stop drug suddenly because this may worsen seizures. Notify prescriber at once if adverse reactions develop.

• Monitor drug levels. Therapeutic level is 10 to 20 mcg/ml.

• Allow at least 7 to 10 days to elapse between dosage changes.

• Monitor CBC and calcium level every 6 months, and periodically monitor hepatic function. If megaloblastic anemia is evident, prescriber may order folic acid and vitamin $B_{12}$.

• Mononucleosis may decrease phenytoin level. Watch for increased seizures.

• Watch for gingival hyperplasia, especially in children.

**Watch out!** Don't confuse phenytoin with fosphenytoin or mephenytoin. Don't confuse Dilantin with Dilaudid.

# pioglitazone hydrochloride
(pigh-oh-GLIH-tah-zohn high-droh-CLOR-ighd)

Actos

Pregnancy risk category: C

## Indications and dosages

**Adjunct to diet and exercise in patients with type 2 diabetes mellitus or when diet, exercise, and a sulfonylurea, metformin, or insulin fail to yield adequate glycemic control**

■ *Adults:* Initially, 15 or 30 mg P.O. once daily. For patients who respond inadequately, dosage may be increased incrementally; maximum dosage, 45 mg daily. If used in combination therapy, maximum dosage shouldn't exceed 30 mg daily.

## Adverse reactions

Aggravated diabetes mellitus • anemia • *edema* • headache • **heart failure** • **hypoglycemia** (with combination therapy) • myalgia • pharyngitis • sinusitis • tooth disorder • upper respiratory tract infection • weight gain

## Nursing considerations

■ Drug is contraindicated in patients with type 1 diabetes mellitus, clinical evidence of active hepatic disease, ALT level greater than 2½ times the upper limit of normal, or New York Heart Association Class III or IV heart failure.

■ Drug is contraindicated in patients with diabetic ketoacidosis and in those who experienced jaundice while taking troglitazone.

*Alert:* Measure liver enzyme levels at start of therapy, every 2 months for first year of therapy, and periodically thereafter. Obtain liver function test results in patients who develop signs and symptoms of hepatic dysfunction, such as nausea, vomiting, abdominal pain, fatigue, anorexia, or dark urine. Stop drug if patient develops jaundice or if liver function test results show ALT level greater than 3 times the upper limit of normal.

■ Pioglitazone alone or with insulin can cause fluid retention that may lead to or worsen heart failure.

■ Because ovulation may resume in premenopausal, anovulatory women with insulin resistance, recommend use of additional contraceptive measures.

■ Watch for hypoglycemia, especially in patients receiving combination therapy.

■ Monitor blood glucose level regularly, especially during situations of increased stress, such as infection, fever, surgery, and trauma.

■ Check blood glucose level and glycosylated hemoglobin periodically to evaluate therapeutic response to drug.

**Watch out!** Don't confuse pioglitazone with rosiglitazone.

# polyethylene glycol and electrolyte solution
(pol-ee-ETH-ih-leen GLIGH-kohl and
ee-LEK-troh-light soh-LOO-shun)

CoLyte, Go-Evac, GoLYTELY, MiraLax, NuLYTELY, OCL

Pregnancy risk category: C

## Indications and dosages

**Bowel preparation before GI examination**

■ *Adults:* 240 ml P.O. q 10 minutes until 4 L are consumed or until watery stool is clear. Typically, give 4 hours before examination, allowing 3 hours for drinking and 1 hour for bowel evacuation.

## Adverse reactions

*Abdominal fullness* ▪ allergic reaction ▪ anal irritation ▪ *bloating* ▪ *cramps* ▪ dermatitis ▪ *nausea* ▪ rhinorrhea ▪ urticaria ▪ *vomiting*

## Nursing considerations

■ Drug is contraindicated in patients with GI obstruction or perforation, gastric retention, toxic colitis, or megacolon.
■ Use tap water to reconstitute powder. Shake vigorously to dissolve all powder. Refrigerate reconstituted solution, but use within 48 hours.

**Alert:** Don't add flavoring or additional ingredients to solution or give chilled solution. Hypothermia has been reported after ingestion of large amounts of chilled solution
■ Give solution early in the morning if patient is scheduled for a midmorning examination. Oral solution induces diarrhea (onset 30 to 60 minutes) that rapidly cleans the bowel, usually within 4 hours.
■ When using to prepare for barium enema, give solution the evening before the examination to avoid interfering with barium coating of colonic mucosa.
■ If given to semiconscious patient or to patient with impaired gag reflex, be sure to prevent aspiration.
■ Patient preparation for barium enema may be less satisfactory with this solution because it may interfere with the barium coating of the colonic mucosa using the double-contrast technique.

## potassium chloride (puh-TAS-ee-um KLOR-ighd)

Apo-K, Cena-K, Gen-K, K+8, K-10, K+ 10, Kaochlor, Kaochlor S-F, Kaon-Cl, Kaon-Cl-10, Kaon-Cl 20%, Kay Ciel, K+ Care, K-Dur 10, K-Dur 20, K-Lease, K-Lor, Klor- Con, Klor-Con 8, Klor-Con 10, Klor-Con/25, Klorvess, Klotrix, K-Lyte/Cl, K-Norm, K-Tab, K-Vescent Potassium Chloride, Micro-K Extencaps, Micro-K 10 Extencaps, Micro-K LS, Potasalan, Rum-K, Slow-K, Ten-K

Pregnancy risk category: C

### Indications and dosages

**To prevent hypokalemia**

■ *Adults and children:* Initially, 20 mEq P.O. daily in divided doses. Adjust dosage p.r.n. based on potassium levels.

**Hypokalemia**

■ *Adults and children:* 40 to 100 mEq P.O. in two to four divided doses daily. Maximum dosage of diluted I.V. potassium chloride is 40 mEq/L at 10 mEq/hour. Don't exceed 150 mEq daily in adults and 3 mEq/kg daily in children. Further doses are based on potassium levels and blood pH.

**Severe hypokalemia**

■ *Adults and children:* Dilute potassium chloride in a suitable I.V. solution of less than 80 mEq/L, and give at no more than 40 mEq/hour. Further doses are based on potassium level. Don't exceed 150 mEq I.V. daily in adults and 3 mEq/kg I.V. daily or 40 mEq/m² I.V. daily in children.

### Off-label use

**Acute MI**

■ *Adults:* For high dose, 80 mEq/L at 1.5 ml/kg/hour for 24 hours with an I.V. infusion of 25% dextrose and 50 units/L regular insulin. For low dose, 40 mEq/L at 1 ml/kg/hour for 24 hours, with an I.V. infusion of 10% dextrose and 20 units/L regular insulin.

### Adverse reactions

Abdominal pain • *arrhythmias* • *cardiac arrest* • confusion • diarrhea • ECG changes • flaccid paralysis • *heart block* • *hyperkalemia* • hypotension • listlessness • nausea • paresthesia of limbs • *postinfusion phlebitis* • *respiratory paralysis* • weakness or heaviness of limbs • vomiting

### Nursing considerations

■ Drug is contraindicated in patients with severe renal impairment; untreated Addison's disease; or acute dehydration, heat cramps, hyperkalemia, hyperkalemic form of familial periodic paralysis, or other conditions linked to extensive tissue breakdown.
■ Give I.V. potassium replacement only with monitoring of ECG and potassium level.
*Alert:* When giving parenterally, give by I.V. infusion only, never I.V. push or I.M. Give slowly as dilute solution; potentially fatal hyperkalemia may result from too-rapid infusion.

# pravastatin sodium
(PRAH-vuh-stat-in SOH-dee-um)

Pravachol

Pregnancy risk category: X

## Indications and dosages

**Primary and secondary prevention of coronary events; hyperlipidemia**
■ *Adults:* Initially, 40 mg P.O. once daily at the same time each day, with or without food. Adjust dosage q 4 weeks, based on patient tolerance and response. Maximum dosage, 80 mg daily.
**Heterozygous familial hypercholesterolemia**
■ *Adolescents ages 14 to 18:* 40 mg P.O. once daily.
■ *Children ages 8 to 13:* 20 mg P.O. once daily.
*Adjust-a-dose:* For patients with renal or hepatic dysfunction, start with 10 mg P.O. daily. For patients taking immunosuppressants, begin with 10 mg P.O. at bedtime and adjust to higher dosages with caution. Most patients treated with combination of immunosuppressants and pravastatin receive up to 20 mg pravastatin daily.

## Adverse reactions

Abdominal pain ▪ chest pain ▪ common cold ▪ constipation ▪ cough ▪ diarrhea ▪ dizziness ▪ fatigue ▪ flatulence ▪ flulike symptoms ▪ headache ▪ heartburn ▪ influenza ▪ *localized muscle pain* ▪ myalgia ▪ myopathy ▪ myositis ▪ nausea ▪ rash ▪ **rhabdomyolysis** ▪ **renal failure caused by myoglobinuria** ▪ rhinitis ▪ urinary abnormality ▪ vomiting

## Nursing considerations

■ Drug is contraindicated in patients with active hepatic disease or conditions that cause unexplained, persistent elevations of transaminase levels.
■ Drug is contraindicated in pregnant and breast-feeding women and in women of childbearing age.
■ Use only after diet and other nondrug therapies prove ineffective. Patients should follow a standard low-cholesterol diet during therapy.
■ Obtain liver function test results at start of therapy and periodically thereafter. A liver biopsy may be performed if elevated liver enzyme levels persist.
**Watch out!** Don't confuse Pravachol with Prevacid or propranolol.

## prednisone (PRED-nih-sohn)

Apo-Prednisone†, Deltasone, Liquid Pred, Meticorten, Orasone, Panasol-S, Prednicen-M, Prednisone Intensol, Sterapred, Winpred†

Pregnancy risk category: C

### Indications and dosages

**Severe inflammation, immuno-suppression**

■ *Adults:* 5 to 60 mg P.O. daily in single dose or as two to four divided doses. Maintenance dose given once daily or every other day; dosage must be individualized.

■ *Children:* 0.14 to 2 mg/kg or 4 to 60 mg/m$^2$ daily P.O. in four divided doses.

**Acute exacerbations of multiple sclerosis**

■ *Adults:* 200 mg P.O. daily for 7 days; then 80 mg P.O. every other day for 1 month.

### Adverse reactions

Acne ▪ *acute adrenal insufficiency* ▪ *arrhythmias* ▪ cataracts ▪ carbo-hydrate intolerance ▪ cushingoid state ▪ delayed wound healing ▪ edema ▪ *euphoria* ▪ GI irritation ▪ glaucoma ▪ growth suppression in children ▪ headache ▪ *heart failure* ▪ hirsutism ▪ hypercholesterolemia ▪ hyperglycemia ▪ hypertension ▪ hypocalcemia ▪ hypokalemia ▪ increased appetite ▪ increased urine calcium level ▪ *insomnia* ▪ menstrual irregularities ▪ muscle weakness ▪ nausea ▪ osteoporosis ▪ *pancreatitis* ▪ paresthesia ▪ *peptic ulceration* ▪ *pseudotumor cerebri* ▪ psychotic behavior ▪ *seizures* ▪

susceptibility to infections ▪ *thromboembolism* ▪ thrombo-phlebitis ▪ various skin eruptions ▪ vertigo ▪ vomiting

<u>After abrupt withdrawal</u>

Anorexia ▪ arthralgia ▪ depression ▪ dizziness ▪ dyspnea ▪ fainting ▪ fatigue ▪ fever ▪ hypoglycemia ▪ lethargy ▪ orthostatic hypotension ▪ rebound inflammation ▪ weakness

### Nursing considerations

▪ Drug is contraindicated in patients with systemic fungal infections and in those receiving immunosuppressant doses with live virus vaccines.

▪ For better results and less toxicity, give a once-daily dose in the morning.

▪ Unless contraindicated, give oral dose with food when possible to reduce GI irritation. Patient may need medication to prevent GI irritation.

▪ Oral solution may be diluted in juice or other flavored diluent or semisolid food before administration.

▪ Monitor patient's blood pressure, sleep patterns, and potassium level.

▪ Weigh patient daily; report sudden weight gain to prescriber.

*Alert:* After prolonged use, sudden withdrawal may be fatal.

**Watch out!** Don't confuse prednisone with prednimustine, prednisolone, or primidone.

O-R

## propranolol hydrochloride
(proh-PRAH-nuh-lohl high-droh-KLOR-ighd)

Apo-Propranolol†, Inderal, Inderal LA, InnoPran XL, Novopranol†

Pregnancy risk category: C

## Indications and dosages

### Angina pectoris
■ *Adults:* Total daily doses of 80 to 320 mg P.O. when given b.i.d., t.i.d., or q.i.d. Or, one 80-mg extended-release capsule daily. Dosage increased at 3- to 7-day intervals.

### To decrease risk of death after MI
■ *Adults:* 180 to 240 mg P.O. daily in divided doses, t.i.d or q.i.d., beginning 5 to 21 days after an MI.

### Supraventricular, ventricular, and atrial arrhythmias; tachyarrhythmias caused by excessive catecholamine action
■ *Adults:* 1 to 3 mg by slow I.V. push, not to exceed 1 mg/minute. After 3 mg has been given, another dose may be given in 2 minutes; give subsequent doses no sooner than q 4 hours. Maintenance dosage, 10 to 30 mg P.O. t.i.d. or q.i.d.

### Hypertension
■ *Adults:* Initially, 80 mg P.O. daily in two divided doses or once daily for extended-release form. Increase at 3- to 7-day intervals to maximum daily dosage of 640 mg. For InnoPran XL, dosage is 80 mg P.O. once daily at bedtime. Maximum dosage of 120 mg daily.
■ *Children:* 0.5 mg/kg P.O. b.i.d. Increase q 3 to 5 days to a maximum dosage of 16 mg/kg daily.

### To prevent frequent, severe, migraine or vascular headaches
■ *Adults:* Initially, 80 mg P.O. daily in divided doses or 1 extended-release capsule daily. Usual maintenance dosage, 160 to 240 mg t.i.d. or q.i.d.

### Hypertrophic subaortic stenosis
■ *Adults:* 20 to 40 mg P.O. t.i.d. or q.i.d.; or 80 to 160 mg extended-release capsules once daily.

## Adverse reactions

Abdominal cramping • *agranulocytosis* • *bradycardia* • *bronchospasm* • constipation • depression • diarrhea • dizziness • *fatigue* • fever • hallucinations • *heart failure* • *hypotension* • insomnia • *intensification of atrioventricular block* • intermittent claudication • *lethargy* • rash • vomiting

## Nursing considerations

■ Drug is contraindicated in patients with bronchial asthma, sinus bradycardia and heart block greater than first-degree, cardiogenic shock, or overt and decompensated heart failure (unless failure is secondary to a tachyarrhythmia.

**Watch out!** Don't confuse propranolol with Pravachol. Don't confuse Inderal with Adderall, Imuran, Inderide, or Isordil.

## protamine sulfate (PROH-tuh-meen SUL-fayt)

Pregnancy risk category: **C**

### Indications and dosages

**Heparin overdose**

■ *Adults:* Base dosage on venous blood coagulation studies, usually 1 mg for each 90 to 115 units of heparin. Give by slow I.V. injection over 10 minutes in doses not to exceed 50 mg.

### Adverse reactions

*Acute pulmonary hypertension* • *anaphylactoid reactions* • *anaphylaxis* • *bradycardia* • *circulatory collapse* • dyspnea • feeling of warmth • hypotension • lassitude • nausea • pulmonary edema • transient flushing • vomiting

### Nursing considerations

■ Have emergency equipment available to treat anaphylaxis or severe hypotension.
*Alert:* Give slowly by direct I.V. injection. Excessively rapid I.V. administration may cause acute hypotension, bradycardia, pulmonary hypertension, dyspnea, transient flushing, and feeling of warmth.

■ Base postoperative dose on coagulation studies, and repeat PTT 15 minutes after administration.

■ Calculate dosage carefully. One mg of protamine neutralizes 90 to 115 units of heparin, depending on salt (heparin calcium or heparin sodium) and source of heparin (beef or pork).

■ Risk of hypersensitivity reaction is greater in patients who are hypersensitive to fish, in vasectomized or infertile men, and in patients taking protamine-insulin products.

■ Watch for spontaneous bleeding (heparin rebound), especially in dialysis patients and in those who have undergone cardiac surgery.

■ Protamine may act as an anticoagulant in very high doses.
**Watch out!** Don't confuse protamine with Protopam or Protropin.

# quetiapine fumarate
(KWET-ee-uh-peen FYOO-muh-rayt)

Seroquel

Pregnancy risk category: C

## Indications and dosages
### To manage signs and symptoms of psychotic disorders
■ *Adults:* Initially, 25 mg PO, b.i.d., with increases in increments of 25 to 50 mg b.i.d. or t.i.d. on days 2 and 3, as tolerated. Target range is 300 to 400 mg daily divided into two or three doses by day 4. Further dosage adjustments, if indicated, should occur at intervals of not less than 2 days. Dosage can be increased or decreased by 25 to 50 mg b.i.d. Antipsychotic effect generally occurs at 150 to 750 mg daily. Safety of dosages over 800 mg daily hasn't been evaluated.
■ *Elderly patients:* Give lower dosages, adjust more slowly, and monitor patient carefully in first dosing period.

### Monotherapy and adjunct therapy with lithium or divalproex for short-term treatment of acute manic episodes associated with bipolar I disorder
■ *Adults:* Initially, 50 mg PO, b.i.d. Increase dosage in increments of 100 mg daily in two divided doses up to 200 mg PO, b.i.d. on day 4. May increase dosage in increments no greater than 200 mg daily up to 800 mg daily by day 6. Usual dosage, 400 to 800 mg daily.
■ *Elderly patients:* Give lower dosages, adjust more slowly, and monitor patient carefully in first dosing period.

*Adjust-a-dose:* For debilitated patients and those with hypotension, consider lower dosages and slower adjustment. For patients with hepatic impairment, initial dosage is 25 mg daily. Increase in increments of 25 to 50 mg daily to an effective dosage.

## Adverse reactions
Abdominal pain • anorexia • asthenia • back pain • constipation • diaphoresis • *dizziness* • dry mouth • dysarthria • dyspepsia • dyspnea • ear pain • flulike syndrome • *headache* • hyperglycemia • hypertonia • increased cough • *leukopenia* • *neuroleptic malignant syndrome* • orthostatic hypotension • palpitations • peripheral edema • pharyngitis • rash • rhinitis • *seizures* • *somnolence* • tachycardia • *weight gain*

## Nursing considerations
*Alert:* Watch for evidence of neuroleptic malignant syndrome, which is rare but commonly fatal. It may not be related to length of drug use or type of neuroleptic; more than 60% of affected patients are men.
■ Monitor patient for tardive dyskinesia, which may occur after prolonged use.

# quinapril hydrochloride
(KWIN-eh-pril high-droh-KLOR-ighd)

Accupril

Pregnancy risk category: C; D in second
and third trimesters

## Indications and dosages

### Hypertension
■ *Adults:* Initially, 10 to 20 mg P.O.
daily. Dosage may be adjusted based
on patient response at intervals of
about 2 weeks. Most patients are
controlled at 20, 40, or 80 mg daily
as a single dose or in two divided
doses. If patient is taking a diuretic,
start therapy with 5 mg daily.
■ *Adult patients older than age 65:*
Start therapy at 10 mg P.O. daily.
*Adjust-a-dose:* For adults with
creatinine clearance over 60 ml/
minute, initially, 10 mg maximum
daily; for clearance of 30 to 60 ml/
minute, 5 mg; for clearance of 10 to
30 ml/minute, 2.5 mg.

### Heart failure
■ *Adults:* Initially, 5 mg P.O. b.i.d. if
patient is taking a diuretic and 10 to
20 mg P.O. b.i.d. if patient isn't taking a diuretic. Dosage may be increased at weekly intervals. Usual
effective dosage, 20 to 40 mg daily
in two equally divided doses.
*Adjust-a-dose:* For patients with creatinine clearance over 30 ml/minute,
first dose, 5 mg daily; if clearance is
10 to 30 ml/minute, 2.5 mg.

## Adverse reactions

Abdominal pain • angina pectoris
• constipation • cough • depression • diaphoresis • diarrhea •
dizziness • dry mouth • fatigue •
headache • *hemorrhage* • *hyperkalemia* • *hypertensive crisis* •
nausea • nervousness • orthostatic hypotension • palpitations •
photosensitivity • pruritus • rhythm
disturbances • somnolence •
tachycardia • vertigo • vomiting

## Nursing considerations

■ Drug is contraindicated in patients
with history of angioedema related
to treatment with ACE inhibitors.
■ Assess renal and hepatic function
before and during therapy.
■ Monitor blood pressure for effectiveness of therapy.
■ Monitor potassium level.
■ Although ACE inhibitors, such as
quinapril, reduce blood pressure in
all races, they reduce it less in
blacks taking ACE inhibitors alone.
Black patients should take quinapril
with a thiazide diuretic for a more
favorable response.
■ ACE inhibitors appear to increase
risk of angioedema in black patients.
■ Other ACE inhibitors have caused
agranulocytosis and neutropenia.
Monitor CBC with differential
counts before therapy and periodically thereafter.

O-R

## rabeprazole sodium
(rah-BEH-pruh-zohl SOH-dee-um)

AcipHex

Pregnancy risk category: **B**

### Indications and dosages

**Healing of erosive or ulcerative gastroesophageal reflux disease (GERD)**
■ *Adults:* 20 mg P.O. daily for 4 to 8 weeks. Additional 8-week course may be considered, if needed.

**Maintenance of healing of erosive or ulcerative GERD**
■ *Adults:* 20 mg P.O. daily.

**Healing of duodenal ulcers**
■ *Adults:* 20 mg P.O. daily after morning meal for up to 4 weeks.

**Pathologic hypersecretory conditions, including Zollinger-Ellison syndrome**
■ *Adults:* 60 mg P.O. daily; may increase p.r.n. to 100 mg P.O. daily or 60 mg P.O. b.i.d.

**Symptomatic GERD, including daytime and nighttime heartburn**
■ *Adults:* 20 mg P.O. daily for 4 weeks. Additional 4-week course may be considered, if needed.

***Helicobacter pylori* eradication, to reduce the risk of duodenal ulcer recurrence**
■ *Adults:* 20 mg P.O. b.i.d., combined with amoxicillin 1,000 mg P.O. b.i.d. and clarithromycin 500 mg P.O. b.i.d., for 7 days.

### Adverse reactions

Headache

### Nursing considerations

■ In *H. pylori* eradication, clarithromycin is contraindicated in pregnant patients, patients hypersensitive to macrolides, and those taking pimozide; amoxicillin is contraindicated in patients hypersensitive to penicillin.

■ Consider additional courses of therapy if duodenal ulcer or GERD isn't healed after first course of therapy.

■ If *H. pylori* eradication is unsuccessful, do susceptibility testing. If patient is resistant to clarithromycin or susceptibility testing isn't possible, expect to start therapy using a different antimicrobial.

**Alert:** Amoxicillin may trigger anaphylaxis in patients with history of penicillin hypersensitivity.

■ Symptomatic response to therapy doesn't preclude presence of gastric malignancy.

**Alert:** Patients treated for *H. pylori* eradication have developed pseudomembranous colitis with nearly all antibacterial agents, including clarithromycin and amoxicillin. Monitor patient closely.

# raloxifene hydrochloride
(rah-LOKS-ih-feen high-droh-KLOR-ighd)

Evista

Pregnancy risk category: X

## Indications and dosages

**To prevent or treat osteoporosis in postmenopausal women**
■ *Adults:* 60 mg P.O. once daily.

## Adverse reactions

Abdominal pain ▪ *arthralgia* ▪ arthritis ▪ breast pain ▪ chest pain ▪ cystitis ▪ depression ▪ diaphoresis ▪ dyspepsia ▪ endometrial disorder ▪ fever ▪ flatulence ▪ *flulike syndrome* ▪ gastroenteritis ▪ *hot flushes* ▪ increased cough ▪ *infection* ▪ insomnia ▪ laryngitis ▪ leg cramps ▪ leukorrhea ▪ migraine ▪ myalgia ▪ nausea ▪ peripheral edema ▪ pharyngitis ▪ pneumonia ▪ rash ▪ *sinusitis* ▪ UTI ▪ vaginal bleeding ▪ vaginitis ▪ vomiting ▪ weight gain

## Nursing considerations

■ Drug is contraindicated in women with past or current venous thromboembolic events, including deep vein thrombosis, pulmonary embolism, and retinal vein thrombosis; in women who are pregnant, planning to get pregnant, or breastfeeding; and in children.
■ Watch for signs of blood clots. Greatest risk of thromboembolic events occurs during first 4 months of treatment.
■ Stop drug at least 72 hours before prolonged immobilization and resume only after patient is fully mobilized.
■ Report unexplained uterine bleeding; drug isn't known to cause endometrial proliferation.
■ Watch for breast abnormalities; drug isn't known to cause an increased risk of breast cancer.
■ Effect on bone mineral density beyond 2 years of drug treatment isn't known.
■ Use with hormone replacement therapy or systemic estrogen hasn't been evaluated and isn't recommended.

## ramipril (reh-MIH-pril)

Altace

Pregnancy risk category: C; D in second and third trimesters

### Indications and dosages

**Hypertension**
■ *Adults:* Initially, 2.5 mg P.O. once daily for patients not taking diuretics, and 1.25 mg P.O. once daily for patients taking diuretics. Increase dosage p.r.n. based on patient response. Maintenance dosage, 2.5 to 20 mg daily as a single dose or in divided doses.
*Adjust-a-dose:* For patients with creatinine clearance less than 40 ml/minute, give 1.25 mg P.O. daily. Adjust dosage gradually based on response. Maximum dosage, 5 mg daily.

**Heart failure after MI**
■ *Adults:* Initially, 2.5 mg P.O. b.i.d. If hypotension occurs, decrease dosage to 1.25 mg P.O. b.i.d. Adjust as tolerated to target dosage of 5 mg P.O. twice daily.
*Adjust-a-dose:* For patients with creatinine clearance less than 40 ml/minute, give 1.25 mg P.O. daily. Adjust dosage gradually based on response. Maximum dosage, 2.5 mg b.i.d.

**To reduce risk of MI, stroke, and death from CV causes**
■ *Adults age 55 and older:* 2.5 mg P.O. once daily for 1 week; then 5 mg P.O. once daily for 3 weeks. Increase as tolerated to a maintenance dosage of 10 mg P.O. once daily.

*Adjust-a-dose:* For patients who are hypertensive or who have recently had MIs, daily dose may be divided.

### Adverse reactions

Abdominal pain ● amnesia ● anorexia ● anxiety ● arthralgia ● arthritis ● asthenia ● chest pain ● constipation ● cough ● depression ● dermatitis ● diarrhea ● dizziness ● dyspepsia ● dyspnea ● edema ● epistaxis ● fatigue ● gastroenteritis ● headache ● *heart failure* ● hyperglycemia ● *hyperkalemia* ● hypersensitivity reactions ● *hypotension* ● impotence ● increased diaphoresis ● insomnia ● lightheadedness ● malaise ● *MI* ● myalgia ● nausea ● nervousness ● neuralgia ● neuropathy ● orthostatic hypotension ● palpitations ● paresthesia ● photosensitivity reactions ● pruritus ● rash ● somnolence ● syncope ● tinnitus ● tremor ● vertigo ● vomiting ● weight gain

### Nursing considerations

■ Drug is contraindicated in patients with a history of angioedema related to treatment with an ACE inhibitor.
■ Monitor blood pressure regularly for drug effectiveness.
■ Closely assess renal function during first few weeks of therapy.
■ Monitor potassium level.

# ranitidine hydrochloride
(ruh-NIH-tuh-deen high-droh-KLOR-ighd)

Apo-Ranitidine†, Zantac, Zantac-C†, Zantac 75, Zantac 150, Zantac 150 GELdose, Zantac 300, Zantac 300 GELdose

Pregnancy risk category: **B**

## Indications and dosages

**Duodenal and gastric ulcer (short-term treatment); pathologic hypersecretory conditions**

▪ *Adults:* 150 mg P.O. b.i.d. or 300 mg daily at bedtime Or, 50 mg I.V. or I.M. q 6 to 8 hours.

▪ *Children ages 1 month to 16 years:* For duodenal and gastric ulcers only, 2 to 4 mg/kg P.O. b.i.d., up to 300 mg/day.

**Maintenance therapy for duodenal or gastric ulcer**

▪ *Adults:* 150 mg P.O. at bedtime.

▪ *Children ages 1 month to 16 years:* 2 to 4 mg/kg P.O. daily, up to 150 mg daily.

**Gastroesophageal reflux disease**

▪ *Adults:* 150 mg P.O. b.i.d.

▪ *Children ages 1 month to 16 years:* 5 to 10 mg/kg P.O. daily given as two divided doses.

**Erosive esophagitis**

▪ *Adults:* 150 mg P.O. q.i.d. Maintenance dosage, 150 mg P.O. b.i.d.

▪ *Children ages 1 month to 16 years:* 5 to 10 mg/kg P.O. daily given as two divided doses.

**Heartburn**

▪ *Adults and children age 12 and older:* 75 mg Zantac 75 P.O. as symptoms occur, up to 150 mg daily, not to exceed 2 weeks of continuous treatment.

*Adjust-a-dose:* For patients with creatinine clearance below 50 ml/minute, 150 mg P.O. q 24 hours or 50 mg I.V. q 18 to 24 hours.

## Adverse reactions

*Anaphylaxis* ▪ *angioedema* ▪ blurred vision ▪ burning and itching at injection site ▪ headache ▪ jaundice ▪ malaise ▪ vertigo

## Nursing considerations

▪ Drug is contraindicated in patients with acute porphyria.

▪ To prepare I.V. injection, dilute 2 ml (50 mg) ranitidine with compatible I.V. solution to a total volume of 20 ml, and inject over at least 5 minutes. Compatible solutions include sterile water for injection, normal saline, $D_5W$, and lactated Ringer's solutions.

▪ To give drug by intermittent I.V. infusion, dilute 50 mg (2 ml) ranitidine in 100 ml compatible solution and infuse at rate of 5 to 7 ml/minute. Infuse premixed solution over 15 to 20 minutes.

▪ Ranitidine may be added to total parenteral nutrition solutions.

**Watch out!** Don't confuse ranitidine with rimantadine. Don't confuse Zantac with Xanax or Zyrtec.

# repaglinide (reh-PAG-lih-nighd)

Prandin

Pregnancy risk category: C

## Indications and dosages

**Adjunct to diet and exercise in patients with type 2 diabetes mellitus whose hyperglycemia can't be controlled satisfactorily by diet and exercise alone; adjunct to diet, exercise, and metformin; adjunct to diet, exercise, and pioglitazone or rosiglitazone**

■ *Adults:* For patients not previously treated or whose glycosolated hemoglobin (HbA$_{1c}$) levels are below 8%, starting dose is 0.5 mg P.O. about 15 minutes before each meal; time may vary from immediately before to as long as 30 minutes before meals. For patients previously treated with glucose-lowering drugs and whose HbA$_{1c}$ levels are 8% or more, first dose is 1 to 2 mg P.O. with each meal. Recommended dosage range, 0.5 to 4 mg with meals b.i.d., t.i.d., or q.i.d. Maximum dosage, 16 mg daily.

Determine dosage by glucose response. May double dosage up to 4 mg with each meal until satisfactory glucose response is achieved. At least 1 week should elapse between dosage adjustments to assess response to each dose.

Metformin may be added if repaglinide monotherapy is inadequate; no repaglinide dosage adjustment is necessary.

*Adjust-a-dose:* For patients with severe renal impairment, starting dose is 0.5 mg P.O. with meals.

## Adverse reactions

Angina ▪ arthralgia ▪ back pain ▪ bronchitis ▪ constipation ▪ diarrhea ▪ dyspepsia ▪ *headache* ▪ hyperglycemia ▪ *hypoglycemia* ▪ nausea ▪ paresthesia ▪ rhinitis ▪ sinusitis ▪ *upper respiratory tract infection* ▪ UTI ▪ vomiting

## Nursing considerations

■ Drug is contraindicated in patients with type 1 diabetes mellitus or diabetic ketoacidosis.

■ Adjust dosage by glucose level response. May double dosage up to 4 mg with each meal until satisfactory glucose level is achieved. At least 1 week should elapse between dosage adjustments to assess response.

■ Loss of glycemic control can occur when the body undergoes stress, such as fever, trauma, infection, or surgery. Stop drug and give insulin.

■ Hypoglycemia may be difficult to recognize in elderly patients and in patients taking beta-adrenergic blockers.

■ When switching to another oral antidiabetic agent, begin new drug on day after last dose of repaglinide.

# rifaximin (righ-FAX-ih-min)

Xifaxan

Pregnancy risk category: C

## Indications and dosages

**Traveler's diarrhea from noninvasive strains of *Escherichia coli***
■ *Adults and children age 12 and older:* 200 mg P.O. t.i.d. for 3 days.

## Adverse reactions

Abdominal pain • constipation • defecation urgency • fever • flatulence • headache • nausea • rectal tenesmus • vomiting

## Nursing considerations

■ Drug is contraindicated in patients hypersensitive to rifaximin or any rifamycin antibacterial.
■ Don't use drug in patients whose illness may be caused by *Campylobacter jejuni* or *Shigella* or *Salmonella* species.

*Alert:* Don't use drug in patients with blood in their stool, diarrhea with fever, or diarrhea from pathogens other than *E. coli.*
■ Stop drug if diarrhea worsens or lasts longer than 48 hours. Patient may need a different antibiotic.
■ Patients who have diarrhea after antibiotic therapy may have pseudomembranous colitis, which may range from mild to life-threatening.
■ Monitor patient for overgrowth of nonsusceptible organisms.

## risedronate sodium (ri-SEH-droh-nate SOH-dee-um)

Actonel

Pregnancy risk category: C

### Indications and dosages

**To prevent and treat postmenopausal osteoporosis**
■ *Adults:* 5-mg tablet P.O. once daily, or 35-mg tablet once weekly.
**Glucocorticoid-induced osteoporosis in patients taking 7.5 mg or more of prednisone or equivalent glucocorticoid daily**
■ *Adults:* 5 mg P.O. daily.
**Paget's disease**
■ *Adults:* 30 mg P.O. daily for 2 months. If relapse occurs or alkaline phosphatase level doesn't normalize, may repeat treatment course 2 months or more after completing first treatment course.

### Adverse reactions

*Abdominal pain* ▪ amblyopia ▪ anemia ▪ angina pectoris ▪ anxiety ▪ *arthralgia* ▪ asthenia ▪ *back pain* ▪ bone pain ▪ bronchitis ▪ bursitis ▪ cataract ▪ chest pain ▪ conjunctivitis ▪ constipation ▪ CV disorder ▪ cystitis ▪ depression ▪ *diarrhea* ▪ dizziness ▪ dyspnea ▪ ecchymosis ▪ flatulence ▪ gastritis ▪ *headache* ▪ *hypertension* ▪ hypertonia ▪ *infection* ▪ insomnia ▪ leg cramps ▪ myalgia ▪ *nausea* ▪ neck pain ▪ neuralgia ▪ otitis media ▪ *pain* ▪ paresthesia ▪ peripheral edema ▪ pharyngitis ▪ pneumonia ▪ pruritus ▪ *rash* ▪ rectal disorder ▪ rhinitis ▪ sinusitis ▪ skin carcinoma ▪ tinnitus ▪ tooth disorder ▪ *UTI* ▪ vertigo

### Nursing considerations

■ Drug is contraindicated in hypocalcemic patients, in patients with creatinine clearance less than 30 ml/minute, and in those who can't stand or sit upright for 30 minutes after administration.
*Alert:* Give drug with 6 to 8 oz of water at least 30 minutes before first food or drink of the day. Don't allow patient to lie down for 30 minutes after taking drug.
■ Consider weight-bearing exercise along with cessation of smoking and alcohol consumption, as appropriate.
*Alert:* Monitor patient for symptoms of esophageal disease (such as dysphagia, retrosternal pain, or severe persistent or worsening heartburn).
■ Patients should receive supplemental calcium and vitamin D if dietary intake is inadequate. Because calcium supplements and drugs containing calcium, aluminum, or magnesium may interfere with risedronate absorption, separate dosing times.

# risperidone (ris-PER-ih-dohn)

Risperdal, Risperdal M-TAB, Risperdal Consta

Pregnancy risk category: C

## Indications and dosages

### Schizophrenia
■ *Adults:* Initially, 1 mg P.O. b.i.d. Increase by 1 mg b.i.d. on days 2 and 3 to a dose of 3 mg b.i.d. Or, 1 mg P.O. on day 1; increase to 2 mg once daily on day 2, and 4 mg once daily on day 3. Wait at least 1 week before adjusting dosage further. Adjust dosages by 1 to 2 mg. Maximum dosage, 8 mg daily (6 to 8 weeks).

### To delay relapse in schizophrenia
■ *Adults:* Initially, 1 mg P.O. on day 1; increase to 2 mg once daily on day 2, and 4 mg once daily on day 3. Dosage range, 2 to 8 mg daily.

### Monotherapy or in combination with lithium or valproate for 3-week treatment of acute manic or mixed episodes from bipolar I disorder
■ *Adults:* 2 to 3 mg P.O. once daily. Adjust dosage by 1 mg daily. Dosage range, 1 to 6 mg daily.
*Adjust-a-dose:* For elderly or debilitated patients, hypotensive patients, and those with severe renal or hepatic impairment, start with 0.5 mg P.O. b.i.d. Increase dosage by 0.5 mg b.i.d. Dosage increases above 1.5 mg b.i.d. should occur at least 1 week apart. Subsequent switches to once-daily dosing may be made after patient is on a twice-daily regimen for 2 to 3 days at the target dose.

### 12-week schizophrenia therapy
■ *Adults:* Establish tolerability to oral form before giving I.M. Give 25 mg deep I.M. gluteal injection q 2 weeks, alternating injections between the two buttocks. Titrate dose no sooner than q 4 weeks. Maximum, 50 mg I.M. q 2 weeks. Continue oral antipsychotic for 3 weeks after first I.M. injection.

## Adverse reactions

*Abdominal pain* • aggressiveness • *agitation* • anemia • *anorexia* • *anxiety* • arthralgia • chest pain • *constipation* • cough • depression • diarrhea (with I.M. form) • dizziness • dry mouth • *dyspepsia* • edema • *extrapyramidal reactions* • fatigue • fever • *headache* • **hyperglycemia** • hypertension (with I.M. form) • hypoesthesia • increased salivation • *insomnia* • leg pain • *nausea* • **neuroleptic malignant syndrome** • orthostatic hypotension • *parkinsonism* • photosensitivity • *rash* • *rhinitis* • somnolence • **suicide attempt** • syncope • tachycardia • **transient ischemic attack or stroke** • vomiting • weight gain

## Nursing considerations

*Alert:* Monitor blood pressure before and during therapy.
**Watch out!** Don't confuse risperidone with reserpine.

# rosiglitazone maleate
(roh-sih-GLIH-tuh-zohn MAL-ee-ayt)

Avandia

Pregnancy risk category: C

## Indications and dosages

**Adjunct to diet and exercise (as monotherapy) in patients with type 2 diabetes mellitus, or (as combination therapy) with sulfonylurea, metformin, or insulin when diet, exercise, and a single agent don't result in adequate glycemic control**
■ *Adults:* Initially, 4 mg P.O. daily in the morning or in divided doses b.i.d. in the morning and evening. May increase dosage to 8 mg P.O. daily or in divided doses b.i.d. if fasting glucose level doesn't improve after 12 weeks of treatment.
*Adjust-a-dose:* For patients stabilized on insulin, continue insulin dose when rosiglitazone therapy starts. Don't give doses of rosiglitazone greater than 4 mg daily with insulin. Decrease insulin dose by 10% to 25% if patient reports hypoglycemia or if fasting glucose level falls below 100 mg/dl.

## Adverse reactions

Accidental injury ● anemia ● back pain ● diarrhea ● edema ● fatigue ● headache ● hyperglycemia ● sinusitis ● upper respiratory tract infection

## Nursing considerations

■ Drug is contraindicated in patients with New York Heart Association Class III or IV cardiac status unless expected benefits outweigh risks.
■ Drug is contraindicated in patients with active hepatic disease, increased baseline liver enzyme levels (ALT level greater than 2½ times upper limit of normal), type 1 diabetes, or diabetic ketoacidosis, and in those who experienced jaundice while taking troglitazone.
*Alert:* Check liver enzyme levels before therapy starts. Don't use drug in patients with increased baseline liver enzyme levels. In patients with normal baseline liver enzyme levels, monitor these levels every 2 months for first 12 months and periodically thereafter. If ALT level is elevated during treatment, recheck levels as soon as possible. Expect to stop drug if levels remain elevated.
■ Because ovulation may resume in premenopausal, anovulatory women with insulin resistance, recommend use of contraceptives.
■ Check glucose and glycosylated hemoglobin levels periodically to monitor therapeutic response to drug.
■ Monitor patient with heart failure for increased edema.
**Watch out!** Don't confuse rosiglitazone with pioglitazone.

# salmeterol xinafoate
(sal-MEE-ter-ohl zee-neh-FOH-ayt)

Serevent Diskus

Pregnancy risk category: C

## Indications and dosages

**Long-term asthma maintenance; to prevent bronchospasm in patients with nocturnal asthma or reversible obstructive airway disease who need regular treatment with short-acting beta agonists**

■ *Adults and children age 4 and older:* 1 inhalation (50 mcg) q 12 hours, morning and evening.

**To prevent exercise-induced bronchospasm**

■ *Adults and children ages 4 and older:* 1 inhalation (50 mcg) at least 30 minutes before exercise. Additional doses shouldn't be taken for at least 12 hours.

**COPD**

■ *Adults:* 1 inhalation (50 mcg) b.i.d. in the morning and evening, about 12 hours apart.

## Adverse reactions

***Bronchospasm*** • cough • diarrhea • dizziness • giddiness • headache • heartburn • hypersensitivity reaction • joint and back pain • lower respiratory tract infection • myalgia • nasal cavity or sinus disorder • *nasopharyngitis* • nausea • nervousness • palpitations • pharyngitis • sinus headache • tachycardia • tremor • *upper respiratory tract infection* • **ventricular arrhythmias** • vomiting

## Nursing considerations

☐ Drug isn't indicated for acute bronchospasm.
*Alert:* Monitor patient for rash and urticaria, which may signal a hypersensitivity reaction.
**Watch out!** Don't confuse Serevent with Serentil.

# sertraline hydrochloride
(SER-truh-leen high-droh-KLOR-ighd)

Zoloft

Pregnancy risk category: C

## Indications and dosages

**Depression**
- *Adults:* 50 mg PO. daily. Adjust dosage p.r.n. and as tolerated. Dosage range, 50 to 200 mg daily.

**Obsessive-compulsive disorder**
- *Adults:* 50 mg PO. once daily. May increase dosage, up to 200 mg daily.
- *Children ages 6 to 17:* Initially, 25 mg PO. daily in children ages 6 to 12, or 50 mg PO. daily in children ages 13 to 17. May increase dosage, p.r.n., up to 200 mg daily at intervals of no less than 1 week.

**Panic disorder**
- *Adults:* Initially, 25 mg PO. daily. After 1 week, increase dosage to 50 mg PO. daily. May increase dosage up to 200 mg daily.

**Posttraumatic stress disorder**
- *Adults:* Initially, 25 mg PO. once daily. Increase dosage to 50 mg PO. once daily after 1 week. May increase dosage at weekly intervals up to 200 mg daily.

**Premenstrual dysphoric disorder**
- *Adults:* Initially, 50 mg PO. daily either continuously or only during luteal phase of menstrual cycle. May increase dosage 50 mg per menstrual cycle, up to 150 mg daily for dosing throughout the cycle or 100 mg daily for luteal-phase dosing. If a 100-mg daily dose has been established with luteal-phase dosing, use a 50-mg

daily adjustment for 3 days at the beginning of each luteal phase.

**Social anxiety disorder**
- *Adults:* Initially, 25 mg PO. once daily. Increase dosage to 50 mg PO. once daily after 1 week. Usual dosage range, 50 to 200 mg daily.

## Off-label use

**Premature ejaculation**
- *Adults:* 25 to 50 mg PO. daily or p.r.n.

**Adjust-a-dose:** For patients with hepatic disease, use lower dosages or less-frequent dosing.

## Adverse reactions

- Abdominal pain • agitation • anorexia • anxiety • chest pain • confusion • constipation • diaphoresis • diarrhea • dizziness • dry mouth • dyspepsia • fatigue • flatulence • headache • hot flushes • hypertonia • hypoesthesia • increased appetite • insomnia • loose stools • male sexual dysfunction • myalgia • nausea • nervousness • palpitations • paresthesia • pruritus • rash • somnolence • suicidal behavior • thirst • tremor • twitching • vomiting

## Nursing considerations

- Drug is contraindicated in patients taking pimozide or MAO inhibitors or within 14 days of MAO inhibitor therapy.

# simvastatin (sim-vuh-STAT-in)

Zocor

Pregnancy risk category: X

## Indications and dosages

**To reduce risk of death from CV disease and CV events in patients at high risk for coronary events**

▪ *Adults:* Initially, 20 mg P.O. daily in evening. Adjust dosage every 4 weeks based on patient tolerance and response. Maximum, 80 mg daily.

**To reduce total and LDL cholesterol levels in patients with homozygous familial hypercholesterolemia**

▪ *Adults:* 40 mg daily in evening; or, 80 mg daily in three divided doses of 20 mg in morning, 20 mg in afternoon, and 40 mg in evening.

**Heterozygous familial hypercholesterolemia**

▪ *Children ages 10 to 17:* 10 mg P.O. once daily in evening. Maximum, 40 mg daily.

*Adjust-a-dose:* For patients taking cyclosporine, begin with 5 mg P.O. simvastatin daily; don't exceed 10 mg P.O. simvastatin daily. For patients taking fibrates or niacin, maximum is 10 mg P.O. simvastatin daily. For patients taking amiodarone or verapamil, maximum is 20 mg P.O. simvastatin daily. For patients with severe renal insufficiency, start with 5 mg P.O. daily.

## Adverse reactions

Abdominal pain ▪ asthenia ▪ constipation ▪ diarrhea ▪ dyspepsia ▪ flatulence ▪ headache ▪ *nausea* ▪ upper respiratory tract infection ▪ *vomiting*

## Nursing considerations

▪ Drug is contraindicated in patients with active hepatic disease or conditions that cause unexplained persistent elevations of transaminase levels.

▪ Drug is contraindicated in pregnant and breast-feeding women and in women of childbearing age.

▪ Use drug only after diet and other nondrug therapies prove ineffective. Patient should follow a standard low-cholesterol diet during therapy.

▪ Obtain liver function test results at start of therapy and periodically thereafter. A liver biopsy may be performed if enzyme elevations persist.

**Watch out!** Don't confuse Zocor with Cozaar.

## sumatriptan succinate
(soo-muh-TRIP-ten SUK-sih-nayt)

Imitrex

Pregnancy risk category: C

## Indications and dosages

**Acute migraines**

■ *Adults:* For injection, 6 mg subQ. Maximum dosage, two 6-mg injections in 24 hours, separated by at least 1 hour.

For tablets, 25 to 100 mg P.O., initially. If desired response isn't achieved in 2 hours, may give second dose of 25 to 100 mg. Additional doses may be used in at least 2-hour intervals. Maximum dosage, 200 mg daily.

For nasal spray, give 5 mg, 10 mg, or 20 mg once in one nostril; may repeat once after 2 hours, for maximum daily dosage of 40 mg. A 10-mg dosage may be achieved by giving a 5-mg dose in each nostril.

**Cluster headache**

■ *Adults:* 6 mg subQ. Maximum dosage, two 6-mg injections in 24 hours, separated by at least 1 hour. *Adjust-a-dose:* For patients with hepatic impairment, maximum single oral dose is 50 mg.

## Adverse reactions

Abdominal discomfort • altered vision • anxiety • *atrial fibrillation* • burning sensation • cold sensation • *coronary artery vasospasm* • diaphoresis • diarrhea • discomfort of throat, nasal cavity, or sinuses, mouth, jaw, or tongue • dizziness • drowsiness • dysphagia • dyspnea

(with P.O. route) • fatigue • flushing • headache • heaviness • *injection site reaction* (with subQ route) • malaise • *MI* • muscle cramps • myalgia • nausea • neck pain • numbness • pressure or tightness in chest • tight feeling in head • *tingling* • **transient myocardial ischemia** • unusual or bad taste (with nasal spray) • upper respiratory inflammation (with P.O. route) • *entricular fibrillation* • *ventricular tachycardia* • vertigo • vomiting • *warm or hot sensation*

## Nursing considerations

■ Drug is contraindicated in patients with history, symptoms, or signs of ischemic cardiac, cerebrovascular (stroke), or peripheral vascular syndromes (such as ischemic bowel disease); significant underlying CV diseases, including angina pectoris, MI, and silent myocardial ischemia; uncontrolled hypertension; or severe hepatic impairment.

■ Drug is contraindicated within 24 hours of another 5-HT$_1$ agonist or drug containing ergotamine and within 2 weeks of MAO inhibitor therapy.

■ Use cautiously in women who are or may become pregnant.

■ After subQ injection, most patients experience relief in 1 to 2 hours.

**Watch out!** Don't confuse sumatriptan with somatropin.

# tamoxifen citrate
(teh-MOKS-uh-fen SIGH-trayt)

Nolvadex, Nolvadex-D†, Novo-Tamoxifen†, Tamofen†, Tamone†

Pregnancy risk category: D

## Indications and dosages

**Advanced breast cancer in women and men**
■ *Adults:* 20 to 40 mg P.O. daily; divide and give doses greater than 20 mg per day b.i.d.
**Adjunct treatment of breast cancer in women**
■ *Adults:* 20 to 40 mg P.O. daily for 5 years; divide and give doses greater than 20 mg per day b.i.d.
**To reduce breast cancer occurrence in high-risk women**
■ *Adults:* 20 mg P.O. daily for 5 years.
**Ductal carcinoma in situ after breast surgery and radiation**
■ *Adults:* 20 mg P.O. daily for 5 years.

### Off-label uses

**McCune-Albright syndrome and precocious puberty**
■ *Children ages 2 to 10:* 20 mg P.O. daily. Treat for up to 12 months.
**To stimulate ovulation**
■ *Adults:* 5 to 40 mg P.O. b.i.d. for 4 days.
**Mastalgia**
■ *Adults:* 10 mg P.O. daily for 10 months.

## Adverse reactions

Alopecia ▪ *amenorrhea* ▪ brief worsening of pain from osseous metastases ▪ cataracts ▪ cholesta-sis ▪ confusion ▪ corneal changes ▪ *diarrhea* ▪ **endometrial cancer** ▪ fatty liver ▪ *fluid retention* ▪ headache ▪ **hepatic necrosis** ▪ *hot flushes* ▪ *hypercalcemia* ▪ *irregular menses* ▪ **leukopenia** ▪ *nausea* ▪ **pulmonary embolism** ▪ rash ▪ retinopathy ▪ *skin changes* ▪ sleepiness ▪ **stroke** ▪ temporary bone or tumor pain ▪ **thrombocytopenia** ▪ **thromboembolism** ▪ **uterine sarcoma** ▪ vaginal bleeding ▪ *vaginal discharge* ▪ *vomiting* ▪ weakness ▪ *weight gain or loss*

## Nursing considerations

■ Drug is contraindicated as therapy to reduce risk of breast cancer in high-risk women who also need coumarin-type anticoagulant therapy and in women with history of deep vein thrombosis or pulmonary embolism.
■ Monitor calcium level. At start of therapy, drug may compound hypercalcemia related to bone metastases.
■ Patient should have baseline and periodic gynecologic examinations because of the small increased risk of endometrial cancer.
■ Rule out pregnancy before treatment begins.
■ Patient may initially experience worsening symptoms.

## tamsulosin hydrochloride
(tam-soo-LOH-sin high-droh-KLOR-ighd)

Flomax

Pregnancy risk category: B

## Indications and dosages

### Benign prostatic hyperplasia (BPH)

■ *Adults:* 0.4 mg P.O. once daily, given 30 minutes after same meal each day. If no response after 2 to 4 weeks, increase dosage to 0.8 mg P.O. once daily.

## Adverse reactions

Abnormal ejaculation ▪ amblyopia ▪ asthenia ▪ back pain ▪ chest pain ▪ decreased libido ▪ diarrhea ▪ *dizziness* ▪ *headache* ▪ increased cough ▪ *infection* ▪ insomnia ▪ nausea ▪ orthostatic hypotension ▪ pharyngitis ▪ priapism ▪ *rhinitis* ▪ sinusitis ▪ somnolence ▪ syncope ▪ tooth disorder ▪ vertigo

## Nursing considerations

■ Monitor patient for decreases in blood pressure.
■ Symptoms of BPH and prostate cancer are similar; rule out prostate cancer before starting therapy.
■ If treatment is interrupted for several days or more, expect to restart therapy at 1 capsule daily.
**Watch out!** Don't confuse Flomax with Fosamax or Volmax.

# telithromycin (teh-lith-ROH-my-sin)

Ketek

Pregnancy risk category: C

## Indications and dosages

**Acute bacterial worsening of chronic bronchitis caused by _Streptococcus pneumoniae, Haemophilus influenzae,_ or _Moraxella catarrhalis;_ acute bacterial sinusitis caused by _S. pneumoniae, H. influenzae, M. catarrhalis,_ or _Staphylococcus aureus_**

■ _Adults:_ 800 mg P.O. once daily for 5 days.

## Adverse reactions

Blurred vision • diplopia • difficulty focusing • _diarrhea_ • dizziness • headache • loose stools • nausea • taste disturbance • vomiting

## Nursing considerations

■ Drug is contraindicated in patients hypersensitive to any macrolide antibiotic.

■ Drug is contraindicated in patients with congenital prolongation of the QTc interval or ongoing proarrhythmic conditions (such as uncorrected hypokalemia, hypomagnesemia, or bradycardia) and in those taking class IA antiarrhythmics (such as quinidine or procainamide) or class III antiarrhythmics (such as dofetilide).

■ Use cautiously in breast-feeding women because telithromycin may be present in breast milk.

■ Telithromycin may cause vision disturbances, particularly in women and patients younger than age 40. Adverse vision effects occur most often after first or second dose, last several hours, and sometimes return with later doses. For some patients, symptoms resolve during treatment; for others, they continue until treatment is complete.

■ Patients with diarrhea may have pseudomembranous colitis.

■ Telithromycin may prolong QTc interval. Rarely, an irregular heartbeat may cause patient to faint.

## temazepam (teh-MAZ-ih-pam)

Restoril

Pregnancy risk category: X

### Indications and dosages

**Insomnia**

■ *Adults:* 15 to 30 mg P.O. at bedtime.

*Adjust-a-dose:* For elderly or debilitated patients, administer 15 mg P.O. at bedtime until individualized response is determined.

### Adverse reactions

Anxiety ● blurred vision ● confusion ● daytime sedation ● depression ● diarrhea ● disturbed coordination ● dizziness ● drowsiness ● dry mouth ● euphoria ● fatigue ● headache ● lethargy ● minor changes in EEG pattern (usually low-voltage fast activity) ● nausea ● nervousness ● nightmares ● physical and psychological dependence ● vertigo ● weakness

### Nursing considerations

■ Assess mental status before starting therapy and expect to reduce dosages in elderly patients; these patients may be more sensitive to the drug's adverse CNS effects.

■ Take precautions to prevent hoarding or overdosing by patients who are depressed, suicidal, or drug-dependent and those with a history of drug abuse.

**Watch out!** Don't confuse Restoril with Vistaril.

## terbutaline sulfate (ter-BYOO-tuh-leen SUL-fayt)

Brethine

Pregnancy risk category: **B**

### Indications and dosages

**Bronchospasm in patients with reversible obstructive airway disease**

■ *Adults and children age 12 and older:* 0.25 mg subQ. May repeat in 15 to 30 minutes, p.r.n. Maximum, 0.5 mg in 4 hours.

■ *Adults and adolescents older than age 15:* 2.5 to 5 mg P.O. t.i.d. in 6-hour intervals during waking hours. Maximum, 15 mg daily.

■ *Children ages 12 to 15:* 2.5 mg P.O. t.i.d. in 6-hour intervals during waking hours. Maximum, 7.5 mg daily.

### Adverse reactions

**Arrhythmias** ● diaphoresis ● *dizziness* ● *drowsiness* ● dyspnea ● flushing ● *headache* ● heartburn ● hypokalemia ● *nausea* ● *nervousness* ● *palpitations* ● **paradoxical bronchospasm** (with prolonged use) ● tachycardia ● *tremor* ● *vomiting* ● weakness

### Nursing considerations

■ Give subQ injections in lateral deltoid area.

■ Terbutaline may reduce the sensitivity of spirometry for the diagnosis of bronchospasm.

■ Protect medication from light. Don't use it if it's discolored.

**Watch out!** Don't confuse terbutaline with terbinafine or tolbutamide.

# tetanus toxoid (TET-uh-nus TOX-oyd)

tetanus toxoid, adsorbed; tetanus toxoid, fluid

Pregnancy risk category: C

## Indications and dosages

**Primary immunization**

■ *Adults and children age 7 and older:* 0.5 ml (adsorbed) I.M. 4 to 8 weeks apart for two doses; then give third dose 6 to 12 months after second. Or, 0.5 ml (fluid) I.M. or subQ 4 to 8 weeks apart for three doses; then give fourth dose of 0.5 ml 6 to 12 months after third dose.

■ *Children ages 6 weeks to 6 years:* Although use isn't recommended in children younger than age 7, the following dosage schedule may be used: 0.5 ml (adsorbed) I.M. at ages 2, 4, and 6 months. Give fourth dose between ages 15 and 18 months. Give fifth dose between ages 4 and 6, just before entry into school, if indicated. Diphtheria and tetanus toxoids and acellular pertussis vaccine adsorbed (DTaP) is recommended for active immunization in children younger than age 7.

**Booster dose**

■ *Adults:* 0.5 ml I.M. at 10-year intervals.

**Postexposure prophylaxis**

■ *Adults:* For a clean, minor wound, give emergency booster dose if more than 10 years have elapsed since last dose. For all other wounds, give booster dose if more than 5 years have elapsed since last dose.

## Adverse reactions

Aches • **anaphylaxis** • chills • encephalopathy • erythema • flushing • headache • hypotension • induration • nodule at injection site • malaise • pains • pruritus • **seizures** • slight fever • tachycardia • urticaria

## Nursing considerations

■ Drug is contraindicated in immunosuppressed patients and in those with immunoglobulin abnormalities or severe hypersensitivity or neurologic reactions to toxoid or its ingredients.

■ Drug is contraindicated in patients with thrombocytopenia or other coagulation disorders that would contraindicate I.M. injection, unless the benefits outweigh risks.

■ Determine date of last tetanus immunization.

■ Keep epinephrine 1:1,000 available to treat anaphylaxis.

■ Adsorbed form produces longer immunity. Fluid form provides quicker booster effect in patients previously actively immunized.

■ Document the manufacturer, lot number, date, and name, address, and title of person giving dose on the patient record or log.

**Watch out!** Don't confuse tetanus toxoid with tetanus immune globulin, human. Both drugs may be given in some situations.

# ticlopidine hydrochloride
(tigh-KLOH-peh-deen high-droh-KLOR-ighd)

Ticlid

Pregnancy risk category: **B**

## Indications and dosages

**To reduce risk of thrombotic stroke in patients who have had a stroke or stroke precursors**
■ *Adults:* 250 mg P.O. b.i.d. with meals.

**Adjunct to aspirin to prevent subacute stent thrombosis in patients having coronary stent placement**
■ *Adults:* 250 mg P.O. b.i.d., combined with antiplatelet doses of aspirin. Start therapy after stent placement and continue for 30 days.

## Adverse reactions

Abdominal pain ● *agranulocytosis* ● *allergic pneumonitis* ● anorexia ● arthropathy ● bleeding ● conjunctival hemorrhage ● dark urine ● *diarrhea* ● dizziness ● dyspepsia ● ecchymoses ● flatulence ● hematuria ● hypersensitivity reactions ● *immune thrombocytopenia* ● *intracranial bleeding* ● maculopapular rash ● myositis ● nausea ● *neutropenia ● pancytopenia* ● peripheral neuropathy ● postoperative bleeding ● pruritus ● rash ● *thrombocytopenic purpura* ● urticaria ● vasculitis ● vomiting

## Nursing considerations

■ Drug is contraindicated in patients with severe hepatic impairment, hematopoietic disorders, active pathologic bleeding from peptic ulceration, or active intracranial bleeding.

■ Because of life-threatening adverse reactions, use drug only in patients who are allergic to, can't tolerate, or are unresponsive to aspirin therapy.

■ Obtain baseline liver function test results before therapy.

■ Determine CBC and WBC differentials at second week of therapy and repeat every 2 weeks until end of third month.

■ Monitor liver function test results and repeat if dysfunction is suspected.

■ Although rare, thrombocytopenia can occur. Stop drug in patients with platelet counts of 80,000/mm$^3$ or less. If needed, give methylprednisolone 20 mg I.V. to normalize bleeding time within 2 hours.

# tiotropium bromide
(tee-oh-TROH-pee-um BROH-mighd)

Spiriva

Pregnancy risk category: C

## Indications and dosages

**Maintenance treatment of bronchospasm in COPD, including chronic bronchitis and emphysema**

■ *Adults:* 1 capsule (18 mcg) inhaled orally once daily using HandiHaler inhalation device.

## Adverse reactions

Abdominal pain ▪ allergic reaction ▪ *angina pectoris* ▪ arthritis ▪ candidiasis ▪ cataract ▪ chest pain ▪ constipation ▪ cough ▪ depression ▪ *dry mouth* ▪ dyspepsia ▪ dysphonia ▪ edema ▪ epistaxis ▪ flu-like syndrome ▪ gastroesophageal reflux ▪ glaucoma ▪ herpes zoster ▪ hypercholesterolemia ▪ hyperglycemia ▪ infection ▪ laryngitis ▪ leg pain ▪ myalgia ▪ paresthesia ▪ pharyngitis ▪ rash ▪ rhinitis ▪ *sinusitis* ▪ skeletal pain ▪ stomatitis ▪ *upper respiratory tract infection* ▪ UTI ▪ vomiting

## Nursing considerations

■ Drug is contraindicated in patients hypersensitive to atropine, its derivatives, ipratropium, or components of the product.
■ Drug is for maintenance treatment of COPD and not for acute bronchospasm.
■ Capsules aren't for oral ingestion. Give them only by oral inhalation with HandiHaler device.
■ Watch for evidence of hypersensitivity (especially angioedema) and paradoxical bronchospasm.

# tirofiban hydrochloride
(ty-roh-FYE-ban high-droh-KLOR-ighd)

Aggrastat

Pregnancy risk category: B

## Indications and dosages

**Acute coronary syndrome, with heparin or aspirin, including patients who are to be managed medically and those undergoing percutaneous transluminal coronary angioplasty or atherectomy**
■ *Adults:* I.V. loading dose of 0.4 mcg/kg/minute for 30 minutes; then continuous I.V. infusion of 0.1 mcg/kg/minute. Continue infusion through angiography and for 12 to 24 hours after angioplasty or atherectomy.
*Adjust-a-dose:* If creatinine clearance is less than 30 ml/minute, use a loading dose of 0.2 mcg/kg/minute for 30 minutes; then continuous I.V. infusion of 0.05 mcg/kg/minute. Continue infusion through angiography and for 12 to 24 hours after angioplasty or atherectomy.

## Adverse reactions

*Bleeding* ▪ bleeding at arterial access site ▪ **bradycardia** ▪ **coronary artery dissection** ▪ diaphoresis ▪ dizziness ▪ edema ▪ fever ▪ headache ▪ leg pain ▪ nausea ▪ *occult bleeding* ▪ pelvic pain ▪ **thrombocytopenia** ▪ vasovagal reaction

## Nursing considerations

■ Drug is contraindicated in patients with active internal bleeding or history of bleeding diathesis within the previous 30 days and in those with history of intracranial hemorrhage, intracranial neoplasm, arteriovenous malformation, aneurysm, thrombocytopenia after previous exposure to tirofiban, stroke within 30 days, or hemorrhagic stroke.
■ Drug is contraindicated in patients with history, symptoms, or findings suggestive of aortic dissection; severe hypertension (systolic blood pressure higher than 180 mm Hg or diastolic higher than 110 mm Hg); acute pericarditis; major surgical procedure or severe physical trauma within previous month; or concomitant use of another parenteral glycoprotein IIb/IIIa inhibitor.
■ Dilute injections of 250 mcg/ml to same strength as 500-ml premixed vials (50 mcg/ml) as follows: Withdraw and discard 100 ml from a 500-ml bag of sterile normal saline solution or $D_5W$ and replace this volume with 100 ml of tirofiban injection (from four 25-ml vials or two 50-ml vials), or withdraw 50 ml from a 250-ml bag of sterile normal saline solution or $D_5W$ and replace this volume with 50 ml of tirofiban injection (from two 25-ml vials or one 50-ml vial), to yield 50 mcg/ml.
*(continued)*

## tirofiban hydrochloride (continued)

■ Inspect solution for particulate matter before administration, and check for leaks by squeezing the inner bag firmly. If particles are visible or leaks occur, discard solution.

■ Give heparin and tirofiban through same I.V. catheter. Give tirofiban through same I.V. line as dopamine, lidocaine, potassium chloride, and famotidine. Don't give drug through the same I.V. line as diazepam.

■ Discard unused solution 24 hours after start of infusion.

■ Store drug at room temperature. Protect from light.

■ Monitor hemoglobin level, hematocrit, and platelet count before starting therapy, 6 hours after loading dose, and at least daily during therapy. Notify prescriber if thrombocytopenia occurs.

■ Give drug with aspirin and heparin.

■ Monitor patient for bleeding.
*Alert:* The most common adverse effect is bleeding at the arterial access site for cardiac catheterization.

■ The sheath may be removed during tirofiban infusion, but only after heparin has been stopped and its effects largely reversed.

■ Minimize use of arterial and venous punctures, I.M. injections, urinary catheters, and nasotracheal and nasogastric tubes.

■ When obtaining I.V. access, avoid use of noncompressible sites (such as subclavian or jugular veins).

**Watch out!** Don't confuse Aggrastat with argatroban.

## tolterodine tartrate (tohl-TER-oh-deen TAR-trate)

Detrol, Detrol LA

Pregnancy risk category: C

### Indications and dosages

**Overactive bladder in patients with symptoms of urinary frequency, urgency, or urge incontinence**

▦ *Adults:* 2-mg tablet P.O. b.i.d. or 4-mg extended-release capsule P.O. daily. May reduce dosage to 1-mg tablet P.O. b.i.d. or 2-mg extended-release capsule P.O. daily, based on patient response and tolerance.
*Adjust-a-dose:* For patients with significantly reduced hepatic function or those taking cytochrome P-450 inhibitors, administer 1-mg tablet P.O. b.i.d. or 2-mg extended-release capsule P.O. daily.

### Adverse reactions

Abdominal pain ▪ abnormal vision ▪ accidental injury ▪ arthralgia ▪ back pain ▪ bronchitis ▪ chest pain ▪ constipation ▪ cough ▪ diarrhea ▪ dizziness ▪ *dry mouth* ▪ dry skin ▪ dyspepsia ▪ dysuria ▪ erythema ▪ fatigue ▪ flatulence ▪ flu-like syndrome ▪ fungal infection ▪ *headache* ▪ hypertension ▪ infection ▪ nausea ▪ nervousness ▪ paresthesia ▪ pharyngitis ▪ pruritus ▪ rhinitis ▪ sinusitis ▪ somnolence ▪ upper respiratory tract infection ▪ urinary frequency ▪ urine retention ▪ UTI ▪ vertigo ▪ vomiting ▪ weight gain ▪ xerophthalmia

### Nursing considerations

▦ Drug is contraindicated in patients with uncontrolled angle-closure glaucoma or urine or gastric retention.
▦ Assess baseline bladder function and monitor therapeutic effects.

# topiramate (toh-PEER-uh-mayt)

Topamax

Pregnancy risk category: C

## Indications and dosages

**Adjunct treatment for partial onset seizures or primary generalized tonic-clonic seizures; Lennox-Gastaut syndrome in children**

■ *Adults:* Initially, 25 to 50 mg PO. daily; increase gradually by 25 to 50 mg/week until an effective daily dosage is reached. Adjust to recommended daily dosage of 200 to 400 mg PO in two divided doses for partial seizures or 400 mg PO. in two divided doses for primary generalized tonic-clonic seizures.

■ *Children ages 2 to 16:* Initially, 1 to 3 mg/kg daily at bedtime for 1 week. Increase at 1- or 2-week intervals by 1 to 3 mg/kg daily in two divided doses to achieve optimal response. Recommended dosage, 5 to 9 mg/kg daily in two divided doses.

**To prevent migraine**

■ *Adults:* Initially, 25 mg PO. daily in the evening for the first week. Then 25 mg PO. b.i.d. in the morning and evening for the second week. For the third week, 25 mg PO. in the morning and 50 mg PO. in the evening. For the fourth week, 50 mg PO. b.i.d. in the morning and evening.

**Adjust-a-dose:** If creatinine clearance is less than 70 ml/minute, reduce dosage by 50%. For hemodialysis patients, supplemental dialysis doses may be needed to avoid rapid drops in drug level during prolonged dialysis treatment.

## Adverse reactions

Abdominal pain • abnormal coordination • *abnormal vision* • acne • aggressive reaction • agitation • alopecia • amenorrhea • anemia • *anorexia* • apathy • arthralgia • *asthenia* • ataxia • back or leg pain • body odor • breast pain • bronchitis • chest pain • *confusion* • conjunctivitis • constipation • cough • decreased libido • depersonalization • depression • diarrhea • difficulty with concentration, attention, language • *difficulty with memory* • diplopia • *dizziness* • dry mouth • dysmenorrhea • dyspepsia • dyspnea • dysuria • edema • emotional lability • epistaxis • euphoria • eye pain • *fatigue* • fever • flatulence • flulike syndrome • gastroenteritis • *generalized tonic-clonic seizures* • gingivitis • hallucinations • hearing problems • hematuria • hot flushes • hyperkinesia • hypertonia • hypoesthesia • hypokinesia • impotence • increased sweating • insomnia • intermenstrual bleeding • *leukopenia* • leukorrhea • lymphadenopathy • malaise • menorrhagia • mood problems • muscle weakness • myalgia • nausea • nervousness • *nystagmus* • palpita-

(continued)

## topiramate *(continued)*

tions • *paresthesia* • personality disorder • pharyngitis • pruritus • *psychomotor slowing* • psychosis • rash • renal calculi • rigor • sinusitis • *somnolence* • *speech disorders* • stupor • **suicide attempt** • taste perversion • tinnitus • *tremor* • *upper respiratory tract infection* • urinary frequency • urinary incontinence • UTI • vaginitis • vasodilation • vertigo • vomiting • weight gain • *weight loss*

### Nursing considerations

▪ If needed, withdraw anticonvulsant (including topiramate) gradually to minimize risk of increased seizure activity.

▪ Monitoring topiramate level isn't necessary.

▪ Drug may infrequently cause oligohidrosis and hyperthermia, mainly in children. Monitor patient closely, especially in hot weather.

▪ Topiramate may cause hyperchloremic, non–anion gap metabolic acidosis from renal bicarbonate loss. Factors that may predispose patients to acidosis, such as renal disease, severe respiratory disorders, status epilepticus, diarrhea, surgery, ketogenic diet, or drugs, may add to topiramate's bicarbonate-lowering effects.

▪ Measure baseline and periodic bicarbonate levels. If metabolic acidosis develops and persists, consider reducing dosage, gradually stopping the drug, or using alkali treatment.

▪ Drug is rapidly cleared by dialysis. A prolonged period of dialysis may cause low drug level and seizures. A supplemental dose may be needed.

▪ Stop drug and notify physician if patient experiences acute myopia and secondary angle-closure glaucoma.

**Watch out!** Don't confuse Topamax with Toprol-XL.

# trazodone hydrochloride
(TRAZ-oh-dohn high-droh-KLOR-ighd)

Desyrel

Pregnancy risk category: C

## Indications and dosages
### Depression
*Adults:* Initially, 150 mg P.O. daily in divided doses; then increase by 50 mg daily q 3 to 4 days p.r.n. Dosage range, 150 to 400 mg daily. Maximum, 600 mg daily for inpatients and 400 mg daily for outpatients.

## Adverse reactions
Anger • anemia • anorexia • blurred vision • confusion • constipation • decreased libido • diaphoresis • dizziness • drowsiness • dry mouth • dysgeusia • dyspnea • ECG changes • fatigue • headache • hematuria • hostility • hypertension • insomnia • nasal congestion • nausea • nervousness • nightmares • orthostatic hypotension • priapism possibly leading to impotence • rash • syncope • tachycardia • tinnitus • tremor • urine retention • urticaria • vivid dreams • vomiting • weakness

## Nursing considerations
■ Give drug after meals or a light snack for optimal absorption and to decrease risk of dizziness.
■ Record mood changes. Monitor patient for suicidal tendencies and allow only minimum supply of drug.
**Watch out!** Don't confuse trazodone with tramadol.

# triamcinolone (trigh-am-SIN-oh-lohn)

triamcinolone
**Aristocort, Atolone, Kenacort**
triamcinolone acetonide
**Azmacort, Kenaject-40, Kenalog-10, Kenalog-40, Tac-3, Tac-40, Triam-A, Triamonide 40, Tri-Kort, Trilog**
triamcinolone diacetate
**Amcort, Aristocort Forte, Aristocort Intralesional, Clinacort, Kenacort, Triam-Forte, Trilone, Tristoject**
triamcinolone hexacetonide
**Aristospan Intra-articular, Aristospan Intralesional**

Pregnancy risk category: C

## Indications and dosages

**Severe inflammation, immuno-suppression**
■ *Adults:* 4 to 48 mg P.O. daily in single dose or divided doses. Or, 40 to 80 mg I.M. acetonide at 4-week intervals. Or, 1 mg acetonide into lesions. Or, initially, 2.5 to 15 mg acetonide into joints (depending on joint size) or soft tissue; then may increase to 40 mg for larger areas. A local anesthetic is commonly injected with triamcinolone into joint. For triamcinolone hexacetonide, up to 0.5 mg (of 5 mg/ml suspension) intralesional or suble-sional injection per square inch of affected skin. Additional injections based on patient's response. Or, 2 to 20 mg (using 20 mg/ml suspension) via intra-articular injection. Dose may be repeated q 3 to 4 weeks.

**Adrenocortical insufficiency**
■ *Children:* 0.117 to 1.66 mg/kg/day or 3.3 to 50 mg/m$^2$/day P.O. in four divided doses.

**Asthma**
■ *Adults and children age 12 and older:* 2 inhalations t.i.d. or q.i.d. Maximum, 16 inhalations daily.
■ *Children ages 6 to 12:* 1 to 2 inhalations t.i.d. or q.i.d. Maximum, 12 inhalations daily.

## Adverse reactions

Acne ▪ *acute adrenal insufficiency following increased stress or abrupt withdrawal after long-term therapy* ▪ *arrhythmias* ▪ carbohydrate intolerance ▪ cataracts ▪ cushingoid state ▪ delayed wound healing ▪ edema ▪ *euphoria* ▪ GI irritation ▪ glaucoma ▪ growth suppression in children ▪ headache ▪ *heart failure* ▪ hirsutism ▪ hypercholesterolemia ▪ hyperglycemia ▪ hypertension ▪ hypocalcemia ▪ hypokalemia ▪ increased appetite ▪ increased urine calcium level ▪ *insomnia* ▪ menstrual irregularities ▪ muscle weakness ▪ nausea ▪ osteoporosis ▪ *pancreatitis* ▪ paresthesia ▪ *peptic ulceration* ▪ *pseudotumor cerebri* ▪ psychotic behavior ▪ *seizures*

*(continued)*

## triamcinolone *(continued)*

- susceptibility to infections •
***thromboembolism*** • thrombophlebitis • various skin eruptions
- vertigo • vomiting

### After abrupt withdrawal

Anorexia • arthralgia • depression
- dizziness • dyspnea • fainting •
fatigue • fever • hypoglycemia •
lethargy • orthostatic hypotension
- rebound inflammation • weakness

### Nursing considerations

*Alert:* After prolonged use, sudden
withdrawal may be fatal.

■ Drug is contraindicated in patients
with systemic fungal infections and
in those receiving immunosuppressant doses with live virus vaccines.

■ Determine whether patient is
sensitive to other corticosteroids.

■ For better results and less toxicity, give a once-daily oral dose in
the morning with food.

*Alert:* Parenteral form isn't for I.V.
use.

*Alert:* Salt formulations aren't
interchangeable.

■ Don't use 40 mg/ml strength for
intradermal or intralesional use;
don't use 10 mg/ml strength for
I.M. use.

■ Don't use diluents that contain
preservatives; flocculation may
occur.

■ Give I.M. injection deeply into
gluteal muscle. Rotate injection
sites to prevent muscle atrophy.

■ Monitor patient's weight, blood
pressure, and electrolyte level.

■ Monitor patient for cushingoid
effects, including moonface, buffalo
hump, central obesity, thinning
hair, hypertension, and increased
susceptibility to infection.

■ Watch for allergic reaction to tartrazine in patients with sensitivity
to aspirin.

■ Watch for depression or psychotic episodes, especially during high-
dose therapy.

■ Patients with diabetes may need
increased insulin dosage; monitor
blood glucose level.

■ Drug may mask or worsen infections, including latent amebiasis.

■ Unless contraindicated, give low-
sodium diet that's high in potassium and protein. Give potassium
supplements p.r.n.

■ Gradually reduce dosage after
long-term therapy. Drug may affect
patient's sleep.

**Watch out!** Don't confuse
triamcinolone with Triaminicin
or Triaminicol.

## trospium chloride (TROH-spee-um KLOR-ighd)

Sanctura

Pregnancy risk category: C

### Indications and dosages

**Overactive bladder with symptoms of urinary urge incontinence, urgency, and frequency**

*Adults younger than age 75:*
20 mg P.O. b.i.d. taken on an empty stomach or at least 1 hour before a meal.

*Elderly patients age 75 and older:*
Based on patient tolerance; reduce dosage to 20 mg once daily.

*Adjust-a-dose:* If creatinine clearance is less than 30 ml/minute, give 20 mg P.O. once daily at bedtime.

### Adverse reactions

Abdominal pain • *constipation* • dry eyes • *dry mouth* • dyspepsia • fatigue • flatulence • headache • urine retention

### Nursing considerations

▪ Drug is contraindicated in patients with or at risk for urine retention, gastric retention, or uncontrolled angle-closure glaucoma.

▪ Assess patient to determine baseline bladder function, and monitor patient for therapeutic effects.

▪ If patient has bladder outflow obstruction, watch for evidence of urine retention.

▪ Monitor patient for decreased gastric motility and constipation.

▪ Elderly patients typically need reduced dosages because they are at an increased risk for anticholinergic effects.

## valacyclovir hydrochloride
(val-ay-SIGH-kloh-veer high-droh-KLOR-ide)

Valtrex

Pregnancy risk category: B

### Indications and dosages

**Herpes zoster infection (shingles)**
■ *Adults:* 1 g P.O. t.i.d. for 7 days.
*Adjust-a-dose:* If creatinine clearance is 30 to 49 ml/minute, give 1 g P.O. q 12 hours; if clearance is 10 to 29 ml/minute, give 1 g P.O. q 24 hours; if clearance is less than 10 ml/minute, give 500 mg P.O. q 24 hours.

**First episode of genital herpes**
■ *Adults:* 1 g P.O. b.i.d. for 10 days.
*Adjust-a-dose:* If creatine clearance is 10 to 29 ml/minute, give 1 g P.O. q 24 hours; if clearance is below 10 ml/minute, give 500 mg P.O. q 24 hours.

**Recurrent genital herpes in immunocompetent patients**
■ *Adults:* 500 mg P.O. b.i.d. for 3 days, given at the first sign or symptom of an episode.
*Adjust-a-dose:* If creatinine clearance is 29 ml/minute or less, give 500 mg P.O. q 24 hours.

**Long-term suppression of recurrent genital herpes**
■ *Adults:* 1 g P.O. once daily. For patients with a history of nine or fewer recurrences per year, use alternative dose of 500 mg once daily.
*Adjust-a-dose:* If creatinine clearance is 29 ml/minute or less, give 500 mg P.O. q 24 hours; give q 48 hours if patient has nine or fewer recurrences per year.

**Cold sores (herpes labialis)**
■ *Adults:* 2 g P.O. q 12 hours for two doses.
*Adjust-a-dose:* If creatinine clearance is 30 to 49 ml/minute, give 1 g q 12 hours for two doses; if clearance is 10 to 29 ml/minute, give 500 mg q 12 hours for two doses; if clearance is less than 10 ml/minute, give 500 mg as a single dose.

**Long-term suppression of recurrent genital herpes in HIV-infected patients with CD4+ cell count of 100 cells/mm³ or more**
■ *Adults:* 500 mg P.O. b.i.d.
*Adjust-a-dose:* If creatinine clearance is 29 ml/minute or less, give 500 mg P.O. q 24 hours.

### Adverse reactions

Abdominal pain ● arthralgia ● depression ● diarrhea ● dizziness ● dysmenorrhea ● *headache* ● *nausea* ● vomiting

### Nursing considerations

*Alert:* Valacyclovir isn't recommended for use in patients with HIV infection or in bone marrow or renal transplant recipients.
**Watch out!** Don't confuse valacyclovir with valganciclovir.

## valganciclovir (val-gan-SIGH-kloh-veer)

Valcyte

Pregnancy risk category: C

### Indications and dosages

**To prevent CMV disease in heart, kidney, and kidney-pancreas transplantation patients at high risk (donor CMV seropositive or recipient CMV seronegative)**
■ *Adults:* 900 mg (two 450-mg tablets) P.O. once daily with food starting within 10 days of transplantation until 100 days after transplantation.

**Active CMV retinitis in patients with AIDS**
■ *Adults:* 900 mg (two 450-mg tablets) P.O. b.i.d. with food for 21 days; maintenance dose is 900 mg (two 450-mg tablets) P.O. daily with food.

**Inactive CMV retinitis**
■ *Adults:* 900 mg (two 450-mg tablets) P.O. daily with food.
*Adjust-a-dose:* If creatinine clearance is 40 to 59 ml/minute, induction dosage is 450 mg b.i.d.; maintenance dosage is 450 mg daily. If clearance is 25 to 39 ml/minute, induction dosage is 450 mg daily; maintenance dosage is 450 mg q 2 days. If clearance is 10 to 24 ml/minute, induction dosage is 450 mg q 2 days; maintenance dosage is 450 mg twice weekly.

### Adverse reactions

*Abdominal pain* • agitation • *anemia* • aplastic anemia • bone marrow depression • confusion • *diarrhea* • hallucinations • *headache* • hypersensitivity reaction • *insomnia* • local or systemic infection • *nausea* • neutropenia • pancytopenia • paresthesia • peripheral neuropathy • psychosis • *pyrexia* • retinal detachment • seizures • sepsis • thrombocytopenia • *vomiting*

### Nursing considerations

■ Drug is contraindicated in patients hypersensitive to valganciclovir or ganciclovir. Don't use in patients receiving hemodialysis.
■ Use cautiously in patients with cytopenias and in those who have received immunosuppressants or radiation.
■ Make sure to adhere to dosing guidelines for valganciclovir because ganciclovir and valganciclovir aren't interchangeable and overdose may occur.
■ Clinical toxicities include severe leukopenia, neutropenia, anemia, pancytopenia, bone marrow depression, aplastic anemia, and thrombocytopenia.
■ Monitor CBC, platelet count, and creatinine level or creatinine clearance frequently during treatment.
**Watch out!** Don't confuse valganciclovir (Valcyte) with valacyclovir (Valtrex).

S-Z

# valproate sodium (val-PROH-ayt SOH-dee-um)

valproate sodium
**Depacon, Depakene**
valproic acid
**Depakene**
divalproex sodium
**Depakote, Depakote ER, Depakote Sprinkle, Epival†**

Pregnancy risk category: **D**

## Indications and dosages

**Simple and complex absence seizures, mixed seizure types (including absence seizures)**
■ *Adults and children:* Initially, 15 mg/kg P.O. or I.V. daily; then increase by 5 to 10 mg/kg daily at weekly intervals to maximum of 60 mg/kg daily.

**Complex partial seizures**
■ *Adults and children age 10 and older:* 10 to 15 mg/kg Depakote or Depakote ER P.O. or valproate sodium I.V. daily; then increase by 5 to 10 mg/kg daily at weekly intervals, up to 60 mg/kg daily.

**Mania**
■ *Adults:* Initially, 750 mg delayed-release divalproex sodium daily in divided doses. Adjust dosage based on patient response; maximum dosage, 60 mg/kg daily.

**To prevent migraine**
■ *Adults:* Initially, 250 mg delayed-release divalproex sodium P.O. b.i.d. Some patients may need up to 1,000 mg daily. Or, 500 mg Depakote ER P.O. daily for 1 week; then 1,000 mg P.O. daily.

**Adjust-a-dose:** For elderly patients, start at lower dosage. Increase dosage more slowly and with regular monitoring of fluid and nutritional intake, and watch for dehydration, somnolence, and other adverse reactions.

## Adverse reactions

*Abdominal pain* ● abnormal thinking ● *alopecia* ● amnesia ● *anorexia* ● *asthenia* ● ataxia ● back and neck pain ● *blurred vision* ● **bone marrow suppression** ● bruising ● bronchitis ● chest pain ● constipation ● depression ● *diarrhea* ● diplopia ● dizziness ● dyspepsia ● dyspnea ● edema ● emotional upset ● **erythema multiforme** ● fever ● *flulike syndrome* ● headache ● **hemorrhage** ● **hepatotoxicity** ● **hypersensitivity reaction** ● hypertension ● hypotension ● increased appetite ● *infection* ● insomnia ● nausea ● *nervousness* ● nystagmus ● **pancreatitis** ● pet-echiae ● pharyngitis ● photosensitivity ● pruritus ● rash ● rhinitis ● *somnolence* ● **Stevens-Johnson syndrome** ● tachycardia ● tinnitus ● *tremor* ● *vomiting* ● weight gain or loss

*(continued)*

## valproate sodium *(continued)*

### Nursing considerations

■ Drug is contraindicated in patients with hepatic disease or significant hepatic dysfunction and in patients with urea cycle disorders.

■ I.V. use is indicated only in patients who can't take drug orally. Switch patient to oral form as soon as feasible; effects of using I.V. dosage for longer than 14 days are unknown.

■ Dilute valproate sodium injection with at least 50 ml of a compatible diluent. It's physically compatible and chemically stable in $D_5W$, normal saline solution, and lactated Ringer's solution for 24 hours.

■ Infuse drug I.V. over 60 minutes (at no more than 20 mg/minute) with the same frequency as oral dosage.

■ Monitoring of drug level and dosage adjustment may be needed.

■ Obtain liver function test results, platelet count, PT, and INR before starting therapy, and monitor these values periodically.

■ Don't give syrup to patients who need sodium restriction. Check with prescriber.

■ Adverse reactions may not be caused by valproic acid alone because this drug is usually used with other anticonvulsants.

■ When converting adults and children ages 10 and older with seizures from Depakote to Depakote ER, make sure the extended-release dose is 8% to 20% higher than the regular dose previously taken. See manufacturer's package insert for more details.

*Alert:* Don't use Depakote ER in children younger than age 10.

■ Divalproex sodium has a lower risk of adverse GI reactions.

■ Never withdraw the drug suddenly because sudden withdrawal may worsen seizures. Call prescriber at once if adverse reactions develop.

*Alert:* Serious or fatal hepatotoxicity may follow nonspecific symptoms, such as malaise, fever, and lethargy. If these symptoms occur during therapy, notify prescriber at once because patient might be developing hepatic dysfunction, which requires patient to stop taking the drug.

■ Patients at high risk for hepatotoxicity include those with congenital metabolic disorders, mental retardation, or organic brain disease; those taking multiple anticonvulsants; and children younger than age 2.

■ Notify prescriber if tremors occur; a dosage reduction may be needed.

■ Monitor drug level. Therapeutic level is 50 to 100 mcg/ml.

■ Use caution when converting patients from a brand-name drug to a generic drug because breakthrough seizures are possible.

# valsartan (val-SAR-tin)

Diovan

Pregnancy risk category: C; D in second and third trimesters

## Indications and dosages

### Hypertension (used alone or with other antihypertensives)

■ *Adults:* Initially, 80 mg P.O. once daily. Expect to see reduction in blood pressure in 2 to 4 weeks. If additional antihypertensive effect is needed, dosage may be increased to 160 or 320 mg daily, or a diuretic may be added. (Addition of a diuretic has a greater effect than dosage increases beyond 80 mg.) Usual dosage range, 80 to 320 mg daily.

### New York Heart Association class II to IV heart failure in patients intolerant of ACE inhibitors

■ *Adults:* Initially, 40 mg P.O. b.i.d.; increase as tolerated to 80 mg b.i.d. Maximum dosage, 160 mg b.i.d.

## Adverse reactions

Abdominal pain ● *angioedema* ● arthralgia ● back pain ● blurred vision ● cough ● diarrhea ● *dizziness* ● dyspepsia ● edema ● fatigue ● headache ● hyperkalemia ● hypotension ● insomnia ● nausea ● *neutropenia* ● orthostatic hypotension ● pharyngitis ● renal impairment ● rhinitis ● sinusitis ● syncope ● upper respiratory tract infection ● vertigo ● viral infection

## Nursing considerations

■ Watch for hypotension. Excessive hypotension can occur when drug is given with high doses of diuretics.

■ Correct volume and salt depletions before starting valsartan.

# vancomycin hydrochloride
(van-koh-MIGH-sin high-droh-KLOR-ighd)

Vancocin, Vancoled

Pregnancy risk category: C

## Indications and dosages

**Serious or severe infections when other antibiotics are ineffective or contraindicated, including those caused by methicillin-resistant *Staphylococcus aureus, S. epidermidis,* or diphtheroid organisms**
■ *Adults:* 1 to 1.5 g I.V. q 12 hours.
■ *Children:* 10 mg/kg I.V. q 6 hours.
■ *Neonates and young infants:* 15 mg/kg I.V. loading dose; then 10 mg/kg I.V. q 12 hours if child is younger than age 1 week or 10 mg/kg I.V. q 8 hours if older than 1 week but younger than 1 month.
■ *Elderly patients:* 15 mg/kg I.V. loading dose. Subsequent doses are based on renal function and serum drug level.

**Antibiotic-related pseudomembranous *Clostridium difficile* and *S. enterocolitis***
■ *Adults:* 125 to 500 mg P.O. q 6 hours for 7 to 10 days.
■ *Children:* 40 mg/kg P.O. daily in divided doses q 6 hours for 7 to 10 days. Maximum dosage, 2 g daily.

**Endocarditis prophylaxis for dental procedures**
■ *Adults:* 1 g I.V. slowly over 1 to 2 hours, completing infusion 30 minutes before procedure.
■ *Children:* 20 mg/kg I.V. over 1 to 2 hours, completing infusion 30 minutes before procedure.

***Adjust-a-dose:*** In patients with renal insufficiency, adjust dosage based on degree of renal impairment, drug level, severity of infection, and susceptibility of causative organism. Initially, give 15 mg/kg I.V.; adjust subsequent doses p.r.n. One possible schedule is as follows: If creatinine level is greater than 5 mg/dl, give 1 g I.V. q 10 to 14 days. If creatinine level is 1.5 to 5 mg/dl, give 1 g I.V. q 3 to 6 days. If creatinine level is less than 1.5 mg/dl, give 1 g I.V. q 12 hours. Or, if glomerular filtration rate (GFR) is 10 to 50 ml/minute, give usual dose q 3 to 10 days, and if GFR is less than 10 ml/minute, give usual dose q 10 days.

## Adverse reactions

***Anaphylaxis*** ▪ chills ▪ dyspnea ▪ eosinophilia ▪ fever ▪ hypotension ▪ *leukopenia* ▪ nausea ▪ *nephrotoxicity* ▪ *neutropenia* ▪ ototoxicity ▪ pain ▪ *pseudomembranous colitis* ▪ red-man syndrome (with rapid I.V. infusion) ▪ superinfection ▪ thrombophlebitis at injection site ▪ tinnitus ▪ wheezing

## Nursing considerations

■ Use cautiously in patients receiving other neurotoxic, nephrotoxic, or ototoxic drugs; in patients older than age 60; and in those with impaired hepatic or renal function,

*(continued)*

## vancomycin hydrochloride (continued)

preexisting hearing loss, or allergies to other antibiotics. Patients with renal dysfunction need dosage adjustments. Monitor blood levels to adjust I.V. dosage. Normal therapeutic levels of vancomycin are peak, 30 to 40 mg/L (drawn 1 hour after infusion ends) and trough, 5 to 10 mg/L (drawn just before next dose is given).

■ For I.V. infusion, dilute in 200 ml normal saline solution for injection or $D_5W$, and infuse over 60 minutes; if dose is greater than 1 g, infuse over 90 minutes.

■ Check I.V. site daily for phlebitis and irritation. Severe irritation and necrosis can result from extravasation.

■ Refrigerate I.V. solution after reconstitution and use within 14 days.

■ Obtain specimen for culture and sensitivity testing before giving first dose. Because of the emergence of vancomycin-resistant enterococci, reserve use of drug for treatment of serious infections caused by gram-positive bacteria resistant to beta-lactam anti-infectives.

■ Obtain hearing evaluation and renal function studies before start of therapy.

■ Monitor patient's fluid balance and watch for oliguria and cloudy urine.

■ Monitor patient carefully for red-man syndrome, which can occur if drug is infused too rapidly. Signs and symptoms include maculo-papular rash on face, neck, trunk, and limbs and pruritus and hypotension caused by histamine release. If wheezing, urticaria, or pain and muscle spasm of chest and back occur, stop infusion and notify prescriber.

■ Don't give drug I.M.

*Alert:* Oral administration is ineffective for systemic infections, and I.V. administration is ineffective for pseudomembranous *(C. difficile)* diarrhea.

■ Oral preparation is stable for 2 weeks if refrigerated.

■ Monitor renal function (BUN, creatinine and creatinine clearance levels, urinalysis, and urine output) during therapy.

■ Monitor patient for signs and symptoms of superinfection.

■ Have patient's hearing evaluated during prolonged therapy.

# vasopressin (VAY-soh-preh-sin)

Pitressin

Pregnancy risk category: C

## Indications and dosages

### Nonnephrogenic, nonpsychogenic diabetes insipidus

■ *Adults:* 5 to 10 units I.M. or subQ b.i.d. to q.i.d. p.r.n. Or, intranasally in individualized dosages, based on response.

■ *Children:* 2.5 to 10 units I.M. or subQ b.i.d. to q.i.d., p.r.n. Or, in individualized dosages.

### To prevent and treat abdominal distention

■ *Adults:* Initially, 5 units I.M.; give subsequent injections q 3 to 4 hours, increasing to 10 units if needed. Children may receive reduced dosages. Or, for adults, aqueous vasopressin 5 to 15 units subQ at 2 hours before and again at 30 minutes before abdominal radiography or kidney biopsy.

## Adverse reactions

Abdominal cramps ● angina in patients with vascular disease ● **arrhythmias** ● **bronchoconstriction** ● **cardiac arrest** ● circumoral pallor ● cutaneous gangrene ● decreased cardiac output ● diaphoresis ● flatulence ● headache ● **hypersensitivity reaction** ● myocardial ischemia ● nausea ● tremor ● urticaria ● uterine cramps ● vasoconstriction ● vertigo ● vomiting ● water intoxication

## Nursing considerations

■ Drug is contraindicated in patients with chronic nephritis and nitrogen retention.

■ Monitor patient for hypersensitivity reactions, including urticaria, angioedema, bronchoconstriction, and anaphylaxis.

■ Synthetic desmopressin is sometimes preferred because of its longer duration of action and less frequent adverse reactions. Desmopressin also is available commercially as a nasal solution.

■ Drug may be used for transient polyuria resulting from ADH deficiency related to neurosurgery or head injury.

■ Warm vasopressin vial in your hands, and mix solution well before administration.

■ Give with 1 to 2 glasses of water to reduce adverse reactions and improve therapeutic response.

■ Monitor urine specific gravity and fluid intake and output to evaluate effectiveness.

■ Monitor patient's blood pressure twice daily. Watch for excessively elevated blood pressure or lack of response to drug, which may be indicated by hypotension. Also monitor weight daily.

**Watch out!** Don't confuse vasopressin with desmopressin.

# venlafaxine hydrochloride
(ven-leh-FAKS-een high-droh-KLOR-ighd)

Effexor, Effexor XR

Pregnancy risk category: C

## Indications and dosages

### Depression
■ **Adults:** Initially, 75 mg PO. daily in two or three divided doses with food. Increase p.r.n and as tolerated by 75 mg daily q 4 days. For moderately depressed outpatients, usual maximum dosage, 225 mg daily; in some severely depressed patients, dosage may be 375 mg daily. For Effexor XR, 75 mg PO. daily in a single dose. Or, start at 375 mg PO. daily for 4 to 7 days before increasing to 75 mg daily. Dosage may be increased by 75 mg daily q 4 days to maximum of 225 mg daily.

### Generalized anxiety disorder
■ **Adults:** Initially, 75 mg Effexor XR PO. daily in a single dose. For some patients, it may be desirable to start at 375 mg PO. daily for 4 to 7 days before increasing to 75 mg daily. Dosage may be increased by 75 mg daily q 4 days to maximum of 225 mg daily.

### Social anxiety disorder
■ **Adults:** Initially, 75 mg daily Effexor XR in a single dose. Or, start at 375 mg PO. daily for 4 to 7 days before increasing to 75 mg daily. Dosage increase p.r.n. by 75 mg daily q 4 days. Maximum dosage, 225 mg daily.

**Adjust-a-dose:** For patients with renal impairment, reduce daily amount by 25%. For those undergoing hemodialysis, reduce daily amount by 50% and withhold dose until dialysis is completed. For patients with hepatic impairment, reduce daily amount by 50%.

## Off-label use

### To prevent major depressive disorder relapse
■ **Adults:** 100 to 200 mg daily PO. (Effexor) or 75 to 225 mg daily PO. (Effexor XR).

## Adverse reactions
Abnormal dreams • *abnormal ejaculation* • agitation • *anorexia* • anxiety • asthenia • blurred vision • chills • constipation • diaphoresis • diarrhea • dizziness • dry mouth • dyspepsia • flatulence • *headache* • hypertension • impaired urination • impotence • infection • insomnia • nausea • nervousness • paresthesia • rash • somnolence • **suicidal behavior** • tachycardia • tremor • urinary frequency • vasodilation • vomiting • weight loss • yawning

## Nursing considerations
■ Drug is contraindicated within 14 days of MAO inhibitor therapy.
**Alert:** Closely monitor patients for suicidal ideation, especially at beginning of therapy and after dosage adjustments.

# verapamil hydrochloride
(veh-RAP-uh-mil high-droh-KLOR-ighd)

Apo-Verap†, Calan, Calan SR, Covera-HS, Isoptin SR, Novo-Veramil†, Nu-Verap†, Verelan, Verelan PM

Pregnancy risk category: C

## Indications and dosages

**Vasospastic angina (Prinzmetal's or variant angina); classic chronic, stable angina pectoris; chronic atrial fibrillation**
■ *Adults:* Starting dose is 80 to 120 mg P.O. t.i.d. Increase dosage at daily or weekly intervals p.r.n. Some patients may require up to 480 mg daily.

**To prevent paroxysmal supraventricular tachycardia**
■ *Adults:* 80 to 120 mg P.O. t.i.d. or q.i.d.

**Supraventricular arrhythmias**
■ *Adults:* 0.075 to 0.15 mg/kg (5 to 10 mg) by I.V. push over 2 minutes with ECG and blood pressure monitoring. Repeat dose in 30 minutes if no response occurs.
■ *Children ages 1 to 15:* 0.1 to 0.3 mg/kg as I.V. bolus over 2 minutes; not to exceed 5 mg.
■ *Children younger than age 1:* 0.1 to 0.2 mg/kg as I.V. bolus over 2 minutes with continuous ECG monitoring. Repeat dose in 30 minutes if no response occurs.

**Digitalized patients with chronic atrial fibrillation or flutter**
■ *Adults:* 240 to 320 mg P.O. daily, divided t.i.d. or q.i.d.

**Hypertension**
■ *Adults:* 240 mg extended-release tablet P.O. once daily in the morning. If response isn't adequate, give an additional 120 mg in the evening or 240 mg q 12 hours, or an 80-mg immediate-release tablet t.i.d.

## Adverse reactions

Asthenia ■ *atrioventricular (AV) block* ■ *bradycardia* ■ constipation ■ dizziness ■ headache ■ *heart failure* ■ nausea ■ peripheral edema ■ pulmonary edema ■ rash ■ *transient hypotension* ■ *ventricular asystole* ■ *ventricular fibrillation*

## Nursing considerations

■ Drug is contraindicated in patients with severe left ventricular dysfunction, cardiogenic shock, second- or third-degree AV block or sick sinus syndrome (except in presence of functioning pacemaker), atrial flutter or fibrillation and accessory bypass tract syndrome, severe heart failure (unless secondary to verapamil therapy), and severe hypotension.
■ I.V. verapamil is contraindicated in patients receiving I.V. beta-adrenergic blockers and in those with ventricular tachycardia.
■ Give drug by direct injection into a vein or into the tubing of a free-flowing, compatible I.V. solution.

*(continued)*

## verapamil hydrochloride *(continued)*

■ Compatible solutions include $D_5W$, half-normal saline solution, normal saline solution, Ringer's solution, and lactated Ringer's solution. Drug is incompatible with sodium bicarbonate.

■ Give I.V. doses over at least 2 minutes (3 minutes in elderly patients) to minimize the risk of adverse reactions.

■ Monitor ECG and blood pressure continuously in patient receiving I.V. verapamil.

■ Although drug should be taken with food, taking extended-release tablets with food may decrease the rate and extent of absorption but allows smaller fluctuations of peak and trough blood levels.

■ Pellet-filled capsules may be given by carefully opening the capsule and sprinkling the pellets on a spoonful of applesauce. This should be swallowed immediately without chewing, and followed by a glass of cool water to ensure all pellets are swallowed.

■ Patients with severely compromised cardiac function and those receiving beta-adrenergic blockers should receive lower doses of verapamil. Monitor these patients closely.

■ If verapamil is being used to treat supraventricular tachycardia, prescriber may have patient perform vagal maneuvers after receiving drug.

■ Monitor blood pressure at the start of therapy and during dosage adjustments. Assist patient with walking because dizziness may occur.

■ Notify prescriber if signs and symptoms of heart failure, such as swelling of hands and feet and shortness of breath, occur.

■ Monitor liver function test results during prolonged treatment.

**Watch out!** Don't confuse Verelan with Virilon, Vivarin, or Voltaren.

## vitamin K analogue
(VIGH-tuh-min KAY AN-uh-log)

phytonadione
**AquaMEPHYTON, Mephyton**

Pregnancy risk category: C

## Indications and dosages

**Recommended daily allowance**
■ *Men ages 19 and older:* 120 mcg.
■ *Women ages 19 and older, including pregnant and breast-feeding women:* 90 mcg.
■ *Children ages 14 to 18:* 75 mcg.
■ *Children ages 9 to 13:* 60 mcg.
■ *Children ages 4 to 8:* 55 mcg.
■ *Children ages 1 to 3:* 30 mcg.
■ *Infants ages 7 months to 1 year:* 2.5 mcg.
■ *Neonates and infants younger than age 6 months:* 2 mcg.
**Hypoprothrombinemia caused by vitamin K malabsorption, drug therapy, or excessive vitamin A dosage**
■ *Adults:* Depending on severity, 2.5 to 10 mg P.O., I.M., or subQ, repeated and increased up to 50 mg p.r.n.
■ *Children:* 5 to 10 mg P.O. or parenterally.
■ *Infants:* 2 mg P.O. or parenterally.
**Hypoprothrombinemia caused by oral anticoagulants**
■ *Adults:* 2.5 to 10 mg P.O., I.M., or subQ based on PT and INR, repeat if needed within 12 to 48 hours after oral dose or within 6 to 8 hours after parenteral dose. In emergency, 10 to 50 mg slow I.V. at rate not to exceed 1 mg/minute, repeated q 4 hours p.r.n.

**To prevent hemorrhagic disease of newborn**
■ *Neonates:* 0.5 to 1 mg I.M. within 1 hour after birth.
**Hemorrhagic disease of newborn**
■ *Neonates:* 1 mg subQ or I.M. Higher doses may be needed if mother has been receiving oral anticoagulants.
**To prevent hypoprothrombinemia related to vitamin K deficiency in long-term parenteral nutrition**
■ *Adults:* 5 to 10 mg P.O. or I.M. weekly.
■ *Children:* 2 to 5 mg P.O. or I.M. weekly.
**To prevent hypoprothrombinemia in infants receiving less than 0.1 mg/L vitamin K in breast milk or milk substitutes**
■ *Infants:* 1 mg I.M. monthly.

## Adverse reactions

***Anaphylaxis or anaphylactoid reactions*** (usually after too-rapid I.V. administration) • diaphoresis • dizziness • erythema • flushing • pain, swelling, and, hematoma at injection site • rapid and weak pulse • transient hypotension after I.V. administration

## Nursing considerations

*Alert:* I.V. use can cause death; use only when other routes of administration aren't feasible.

*(continued)*

## vitamin K analogue (continued)

Effects of I.V. injection are more rapid but shorter-lived than I.M. or subQ injections.

Dilute with normal saline solution, $D_5W$, or 5% dextrose in normal saline solution for injection.

Give I.V. by slow infusion over 2 to 3 hours. Don't exceed 1 mg/minute.

Protect parenteral products from light. Wrap infusion container with aluminum foil or other dark cover.

Check brand name labels for administration route restrictions.

For I.M. administration in adults and older children, give in upper outer quadrant of buttocks; for infants, give in anterolateral aspect of thigh or deltoid region. SubQ route is preferred to avoid hematoma formation.

Allergic reactions may occur after I.M. or subQ use.

Anticipate order for weekly addition of 5 to 10 mg of phytonadione to total parenteral nutrition solutions.

Monitor PT or INR to determine dosage effectiveness.

If severe bleeding occurs, don't delay other measures, such as administration of fresh frozen plasma or whole blood.

Vitamin K doesn't reverse the anticoagulant effects of heparin.

*Alert:* Watch for flushing, weakness, tachycardia, and hypotension; these symptoms may signal impending shock.

Phytonadione for hemorrhagic disease in infants causes fewer adverse reactions than other vitamin K analogues.

# warfarin sodium (WAR-feh-rin SOH-dee-um)

Coumadin, Warfilone†

Pregnancy risk category: X

## Indications and dosages

**Pulmonary embolism with deep vein thrombosis, MI, rheumatic heart disease with heart valve damage, prosthetic heart valves, chronic atrial fibrillation**

▪ *Adults:* 2 to 5 mg P.O. daily for 2 to 4 days; then dosage based on daily PT and INR. Usual maintenance dosage, 2 to 10 mg P.O. daily; I.V. dosage is same as P.O.

## Adverse reactions

Alopecia ▪ anorexia ▪ cramps ▪ dermatitis ▪ *diarrhea* ▪ enhanced uric acid excretion ▪ excessive menstrual bleeding ▪ *fever* ▪ gangrene ▪ headache ▪ hematuria ▪ ***hemorrhage*** ▪ ***hepatitis*** ▪ jaundice ▪ melena ▪ mouth ulcerations ▪ nausea ▪ necrosis ▪ *rash* ▪ sore mouth ▪ urticaria ▪ vomiting

## Nursing considerations

▪ Drug is contraindicated in patients with bleeding from the GI, GU, or respiratory tract; aneurysm; cerebrovascular hemorrhage; severe or malignant hypertension; severe renal or hepatic disease; subacute bacterial endocarditis, pericarditis, or pericardial effusion; or blood dyscrasias or hemorrhagic tendencies.

▪ Drug is contraindicated during pregnancy, threatened abortion, eclampsia, or preeclampsia and after recent surgery involving large open areas of the eye, brain, or spinal cord.

▪ I.V. form may be ordered in rare instances when oral therapy can't be given. Reconstitute powder with 2.7 ml sterile water or as instructed in manufacturer guidelines. Give I.V. as a slow bolus injection over 1 to 2 minutes into a peripheral vein.

▪ Because onset of action is delayed, heparin sodium is commonly given during first few days of treatment.

▪ Draw blood for PT and INR before and during therapy.

▪ Give warfarin at same time daily. INR range for chronic atrial fibrillation is usually 2 to 3.

▪ Regularly inspect patient for bleeding gums, bruises on arms or legs, petechiae, nosebleeds, melena, tarry stools, hematuria, and hematemesis.

▪ Check for unexpected bleeding in breast-fed infants of women on drug.

**Alert:** Withhold drug and call prescriber at once in the event of fever or rash (signs of severe adverse reactions).

▪ Effect can be neutralized by parenteral or oral vitamin K.

## zafirlukast (zay-FEER-loo-kast)

Accolate

Pregnancy risk category: B

### Indications and dosages

**Prevention and long-term treatment of asthma**
■ *Adults and children age 12 and older:* 20 mg P.O. b.i.d. 1 hour before or 2 hours after meals.
■ *Children ages 5 to 11:* 10 mg P.O. b.i.d. 1 hour before or 2 hours after meals.

### Adverse reactions

Abdominal pain ▪ asthenia ▪ back pain ▪ diarrhea ▪ dizziness ▪ dyspepsia ▪ fever ▪ gastritis ▪ *headache* ▪ infection ▪ myalgia ▪ nausea ▪ pain ▪ vomiting

### Nursing considerations

■ Drug is contraindicated in breast-feeding women.
■ Drug is contraindicated to reverse bronchospasm in acute asthma attacks.
*Alert:* Reduction in oral corticosteroid dosage has been followed in rare cases by eosinophilia, vasculitic rash, worsening pulmonary symptoms, cardiac complications, or neuropathy, sometimes presenting as Churg-Strauss syndrome.

# zolpidem tartrate (ZOHL-peh-dim TAR-trayt)

Ambien

Pregnancy risk category: **B**

## Indications and dosages

### Short-term management of insomnia
■ *Adults:* 10 mg P.O. immediately before bedtime.
■ *Elderly patients:* 5 mg P.O. immediately before bedtime. Maximum dosage, 10 mg daily.
*Adjust-a-dose:* For debilitated patients and those with hepatic insufficiency, 5 mg P.O. immediately before bedtime. Maximum dosage, 10 mg daily.

## Adverse reactions

Abdominal pain ● altered dreams ● amnesia ● arthralgia ● back or chest pain ● constipation ● daytime drowsiness ● depression ● diarrhea ● dizziness ● dry mouth ● dyspepsia ● flulike syndrome ● hangover ● *headache* ● hypersensitivity reactions ● lethargy ● lightheadedness ● myalgia ● nausea ● nervousness ● palpitations ● pharyngitis ● rash ● sinusitis ● sleep disorder ● vomiting

## Nursing considerations

■ Use hypnotics, such as zolpidem, only for short-term management (usually 7 to 10 days) of insomnia.
■ Use the smallest effective dosage in all patients.
■ Take precautions to prevent hoarding or overdosing by patients who are depressed, suicidal, or drug-dependent or who have history of drug abuse.
**Watch out!** Don't confuse Ambien with Amen.

# zonisamide (zon-ISS-a-mide)

Zonegran

Pregnancy risk category: C

## Indications and dosages

### Adjunct therapy for partial seizures in adults with epilepsy

■ *Adults and children older than age 16:* Initially, 100 mg P.O. as a single daily dose for 2 weeks. Then increase dosage to 200 mg daily p.r.n. for at least 2 weeks. Dosage may then be increased to 300 mg and 400 mg P.O. daily, with the dosage stable for at least 2 weeks. Doses can be given once or twice daily except for the daily dose of 100 mg at start of therapy. Maximum dosage, 600 mg daily.

## Adverse reactions

Abdominal pain ● agitation or irritability ● amblyopia ● *anorexia* ● anxiety ● asthenia ● ataxia ● confusion ● constipation ● cough ● depression ● diarrhea ● difficulty with concentration, memory, or verbal expression ● diplopia ● *dizziness* ● dry mouth ● dyspepsia ● ecchymoses ● fatigue ● flulike syndrome ● *headache* ● hyperesthesia ● incoordination ● insomnia ● mental slowing ● nausea ● nervousness ● nystagmus ● paresthe-

sia ● pharyngitis ● pruritus ● rash ● renal calculi ● rhinitis ● schizophrenic or schizophreniform behavior ● *seizures* ● somnolence ● speech disorders ● *status epilepticus* ● taste perversion ● tinnitus ● tremor ● vomiting ● weight loss

## Nursing considerations

■ Drug is contraindicated in patients hypersensitive to sulfonamides.
■ Drug is contraindicated in those with glomerular filtration rates less than 50 ml/minute.
■ If patient develops acute renal failure or a significant sustained increase in creatinine or BUN level, stop drug and notify prescriber.
■ Achieving steady-state levels may take 2 weeks.
■ Don't stop drug abruptly because this may cause increased seizures or status epilepticus; reduce dosage or stop drug gradually, as prescribed.
■ Increase fluid intake and urine output to help prevent renal calculi.
■ Monitor renal function periodically.

**INFUSION RATES**

## Epinephrine and nitroglycerin

### Epinephrine

Mix 1 mg in 250 ml (4 mcg/ml).

| Dosage (mcg/min) | Infusion rate (ml/hr) |
|---|---|
| 1 | 15 |
| 2 | 30 |
| 3 | 45 |
| 4 | 60 |

### Nitroglycerin

Determine the infusion rate in milliliters per hour (ml/hr) using the ordered dose and the concentration of the drug solution.

| Dosage (mcg/min) | 50 mg/250 ml (200 mcg/ml) | 100 mg/250 ml (400 mcg/ml) |
|---|---|---|
| 5 | 2 | 1 |
| 10 | 3 | 2 |
| 20 | 6 | 3 |
| 30 | 9 | 5 |
| 40 | 12 | 6 |
| 50 | 15 | 8 |
| 60 | 18 | 9 |
| 70 | 21 | 10 |
| 80 | 24 | 12 |
| 90 | 27 | 14 |
| 100 | 30 | 15 |
| 150 | 45 | 23 |
| 200 | 60 | 30 |

## Dobutamine

Mix 250 mg in 250 ml of D$_5$W (1,000 mcg/ml). Determine the infusion rate in milliliters per hour (ml/hr), using the ordered dose and the patient's weight in pounds (lb) or kilograms (kg).

| Dose (mcg/kg/min) | Patient's weight | | | | | | | | | | | | | | |
|---|---|---|---|---|---|---|---|---|---|---|---|---|---|---|---|
| | lb 88 | 99 | 110 | 121 | 132 | 143 | 154 | 165 | 176 | 187 | 198 | 209 | 220 | 231 | 242 |
| | kg 40 | 45 | 50 | 55 | 60 | 65 | 70 | 75 | 80 | 85 | 90 | 95 | 100 | 105 | 110 |
| 2.5 | 6 | 7 | 8 | 8 | 9 | 10 | 11 | 11 | 12 | 13 | 14 | 14 | 15 | 16 | 17 |
| 5 | 12 | 14 | 15 | 17 | 18 | 20 | 21 | 23 | 24 | 26 | 27 | 29 | 30 | 32 | 33 |
| 7.5 | 18 | 20 | 23 | 25 | 27 | 29 | 32 | 34 | 36 | 38 | 41 | 43 | 45 | 47 | 50 |
| 10 | 24 | 27 | 30 | 33 | 36 | 39 | 42 | 45 | 48 | 51 | 54 | 57 | 60 | 63 | 66 |
| 12.5 | 30 | 34 | 38 | 41 | 45 | 49 | 53 | 56 | 60 | 64 | 68 | 71 | 75 | 79 | 83 |
| 15 | 36 | 41 | 45 | 50 | 54 | 59 | 63 | 68 | 72 | 77 | 81 | 86 | 90 | 95 | 99 |
| 20 | 48 | 54 | 60 | 66 | 72 | 78 | 84 | 90 | 96 | 102 | 108 | 114 | 120 | 126 | 132 |
| 25 | 60 | 68 | 75 | 83 | 90 | 98 | 105 | 113 | 120 | 128 | 135 | 143 | 150 | 158 | 165 |
| 30 | 72 | 81 | 90 | 99 | 108 | 117 | 126 | 135 | 144 | 153 | 162 | 171 | 180 | 189 | 198 |
| 35 | 84 | 95 | 105 | 116 | 126 | 137 | 147 | 158 | 168 | 179 | 189 | 200 | 210 | 221 | 231 |
| 40 | 96 | 108 | 120 | 132 | 144 | 156 | 168 | 180 | 192 | 204 | 216 | 228 | 240 | 252 | 264 |

# Dopamine

Mix 400 mg in 250 ml of D$_5$W (1,600 mcg/ml). Determine the infusion rate in milliliters per hour (ml/hr), using the ordered dose and the patient's weight in pounds (lb) or kilograms (kg).

| Dose (mcg/kg/min) | lb 88 kg 40 | 99 45 | 110 50 | 121 55 | 132 60 | 143 65 | 154 70 | 165 75 | 176 80 | 187 85 | 198 90 | 209 95 | 220 100 | 231 105 |
|---|---|---|---|---|---|---|---|---|---|---|---|---|---|---|
| | | | | | | Patient's weight | | | | | | | | |
| 2.5 | 4 | 5 | 5 | 5 | 6 | 6 | 7 | 7 | 8 | 8 | 8 | 9 | 9 | 10 |
| 5 | 8 | 8 | 9 | 10 | 11 | 12 | 13 | 14 | 15 | 16 | 17 | 18 | 19 | 20 |
| 7.5 | 11 | 13 | 14 | 15 | 17 | 18 | 20 | 21 | 23 | 24 | 25 | 27 | 28 | 30 |
| 10 | 15 | 17 | 19 | 21 | 23 | 24 | 26 | 28 | 30 | 32 | 34 | 36 | 38 | 39 |
| 12.5 | 19 | 21 | 23 | 26 | 28 | 30 | 33 | 35 | 38 | 40 | 42 | 45 | 47 | 49 |
| 15 | 23 | 25 | 28 | 31 | 34 | 37 | 39 | 42 | 45 | 48 | 51 | 53 | 56 | 59 |
| 20 | 30 | 34 | 38 | 41 | 45 | 49 | 53 | 56 | 60 | 64 | 68 | 71 | 75 | 79 |
| 25 | 38 | 42 | 47 | 52 | 56 | 61 | 66 | 70 | 75 | 80 | 84 | 89 | 94 | 98 |
| 30 | 45 | 51 | 56 | 62 | 67 | 73 | 79 | 84 | 90 | 96 | 101 | 107 | 113 | 118 |
| 35 | 53 | 59 | 66 | 72 | 79 | 85 | 92 | 98 | 105 | 112 | 118 | 125 | 131 | 138 |
| 40 | 60 | 68 | 75 | 83 | 90 | 98 | 105 | 113 | 120 | 128 | 135 | 143 | 150 | 158 |
| 45 | 68 | 76 | 84 | 93 | 101 | 110 | 118 | 127 | 135 | 143 | 152 | 160 | 169 | 177 |
| 50 | 75 | 84 | 94 | 103 | 113 | 122 | 131 | 141 | 150 | 159 | 169 | 178 | 188 | 197 |

I.V.

## Nitroprusside

Mix 50 mg in 250 ml of $D_5W$ (200 mcg/ml). Determine the infusion rate in milliliters per hour (ml/hr) using the ordered dose and the patient's weight in pounds (lb) or kilograms (kg).

| Dose (mcg/kg/min) | lb 88 kg 40 | 99 45 | 110 50 | 121 55 | 132 60 | 143 65 | 154 70 | 165 75 | 176 80 | 187 85 | 198 90 | 209 95 | 220 100 | 231 105 | 242 110 |
|---|---|---|---|---|---|---|---|---|---|---|---|---|---|---|---|
| | | | | | | Patient's weight | | | | | | | | | |
| 0.3 | 4 | 4 | 5 | 5 | 5 | 6 | 6 | 7 | 7 | 8 | 8 | 9 | 9 | 9 | 10 |
| 0.5 | 6 | 7 | 8 | 8 | 9 | 10 | 11 | 11 | 12 | 13 | 14 | 14 | 15 | 16 | 17 |
| 1 | 12 | 14 | 15 | 17 | 18 | 20 | 21 | 23 | 24 | 26 | 27 | 29 | 30 | 32 | 33 |
| 1.5 | 18 | 20 | 23 | 25 | 27 | 29 | 32 | 34 | 36 | 38 | 41 | 43 | 45 | 47 | 50 |
| 2 | 24 | 27 | 30 | 33 | 36 | 39 | 42 | 45 | 48 | 51 | 54 | 57 | 60 | 63 | 66 |
| 3 | 36 | 41 | 45 | 50 | 54 | 59 | 63 | 68 | 72 | 77 | 81 | 86 | 90 | 95 | 99 |
| 4 | 48 | 54 | 60 | 66 | 72 | 78 | 84 | 90 | 96 | 102 | 108 | 114 | 120 | 126 | 132 |
| 5 | 60 | 68 | 75 | 83 | 90 | 98 | 105 | 113 | 120 | 128 | 135 | 143 | 150 | 158 | 165 |
| 6 | 72 | 81 | 90 | 99 | 108 | 117 | 126 | 135 | 144 | 153 | 162 | 171 | 180 | 189 | 198 |
| 7 | 84 | 95 | 105 | 116 | 126 | 137 | 147 | 158 | 168 | 179 | 189 | 200 | 210 | 221 | 231 |
| 8 | 96 | 108 | 120 | 132 | 144 | 156 | 168 | 180 | 192 | 204 | 216 | 228 | 240 | 252 | 264 |
| 9 | 108 | 122 | 135 | 149 | 162 | 176 | 189 | 203 | 216 | 230 | 243 | 257 | 270 | 284 | 297 |
| 10 | 120 | 135 | 150 | 165 | 180 | 195 | 210 | 225 | 240 | 255 | 270 | 285 | 300 | 315 | 330 |

## Phenylephrine and norepinephrine

**Phenylephrine**
Mix 25 mg in 250 ml (100 mcg/ml).

| Infusion Rate (ml/hr) | Dosage (mcg/min) |
|---|---|
| 10 | 16 |
| 20 | 32 |
| 30 | 48 |
| 40 | 64 |
| 50 | 80 |
| 60 | 96 |
| 70 | 112 |
| 80 | 128 |
| 90 | 144 |
| 100 | 160 |
| 110 | 176 |
| 120 | 192 |

**Norepinephrine**
Mix 8 mg in 500 ml (16 mcg/ml).

| Infusion Rate (ml/hr) | Dosage (mcg/min) |
|---|---|
| 10 | 3 |
| 15 | 4 |
| 20 | 5 |
| 25 | 7 |
| 30 | 8 |
| 35 | 9 |
| 40 | 11 |
| 45 | 12 |
| 50 | 13 |
| 55 | 15 |
| 60 | 16 |
| 65 | 17 |
| 70 | 19 |
| 75 | 20 |

## Common antidotes

| Drug or toxin | Antidote |
| --- | --- |
| Acetaminophen | Acetylcysteine (Mucomyst) |
| Anticholinergics | Physostigmine (Antilirium) |
| Benzodiazepines | Flumazenil (Romazicon) |
| Calcium channel blockers | Calcium chloride |
| Cyanide | Amyl nitrate, sodium nitrate, and sodium thiosulfate (Cyanide Antidote Kit); methylene blue |
| Digoxin, cardiac glycosides | Digoxin immune fab (Digibind) |
| Heparin | Protamine sulfate |
| Iron | Deferoxamine mesylate (Desferal) |
| Lead | Edetate calcium disodium (Calcium Disodium Versenate) |
| Opioids | Naloxone (Narcan), nalmefene (Revex), naltrexone (ReVia) |
| Organophosphates, anticholinesterases | Atropine, pralidoxime (Protopam) |
| Warfarin | Vitamin K |

# Bradycardia algorithm

**Bradycardia**
- Slow (absolute bradycardia = rate < 60 beats/min)
- Relatively slow (rate less than expected)

*Primary ABCD survey*
- Assess ABCs.
- Secure airway noninvasively.
- Ensure that monitor or defibrillator is available.

*Secondary ABCD survey*
- Secondary ABCs (invasive airway)
- Oxygen, I.V. access, monitor fluids
- Vital signs, pulse oximetry, blood pressure
- 12-lead ECG, portable chest X-ray
- Problem-focused history and physical examination
- Differential diagnoses

Serious signs or symptoms?
Due to bradycardia?

**No**

Type II second-degree AV block
or third-degree AV block?

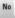

**No**

Monitor the patient.

**Yes**

- Prepare for transvenous pacer.
- If symptoms develop, use transcutaneous pacemaker until transvenous pacer is placed.

**Yes**

*Intervention sequence*
- Atropine I.V. bolus
- Transcutaneous pacing
- Dopamine I.V. infusion
- Epinephrine I.V. infusion
- Isoproterenol I.V. infusion

## Narrow-complex tachycardia algorithm

| Narrow-complex tachycardia, stable |
| --- |

*Therapeutic diagnostic maneuvers*
• Vagal stimulation    • Adenosine

**Junctional tachycardia**

**Preserved**
• Beta-adrenergic blocker
• Calcium channel blocker
• Amiodarone
• No cardioversion

**Impaired***
• Amiodarone
• No cardioversion

**Paroxysmal supraventricular tachycardia**

**Preserved**
*Treatments (in order)*
• Beta-adrenergic blocker
• Calcium channel blocker
• Digoxin
• Cardioversion
• Consider procainamide, amiodarone, sotalol

**Impaired***
*Treatments (in order)*
• Cardioversion
• Digoxin
• Amiodarone
• Diltiazem

**Ectopic beats or multifocal atrial tachycardia**

**Preserved**
• Beta-adrenergic blocker
• Calcium channel blocker
• Amiodarone
• No cardioversion

**Impaired***
• Amiodarone
• Diltiazem
• No cardioversion

*Impaired = ejection fraction < 40%, heart failure

# VF and pulseless VT algorithm

**Primary ABCD survey**
*Focus: Basic CPR and defibrillation*

- Check responsiveness.
- Activate emergency response system.
- Call for defibrillator.
- **A**irway: Open the airway.
- **B**reathing: Provide positive-pressure ventilations.

- **C**irculation: Give chest compressions.
- **D**efibrillation: Monitor for VF or pulseless VT; defibrillate up to three times (200 joules, 200 to 300 joules, 360 joules, or equivalent biphasic).

Rhythm after first three shocks?

Persistent or recurrent VF or VT

**Secondary ABCD survey**
*Focus: Advanced assessments and treatments*

- **A**irway: Insert and secure airway device.
- **B**reathing: Confirm airway device placement and effective oxygenation and ventilation.

- **C**irculation: Establish I.V. access. Monitor rhythm. Administer appropriate drugs.
- **D**ifferential diagnosis.

- Epinephrine I.V. push; repeat every 3 to 5 min **or**  • Vasopressin I.V.; single dose only

Resume attempts to defibrillate: 1 × 360 joules within 30 to 60 sec

*Consider antiarrhythmics:*
- Amiodarone        • Lidocaine        • Magnesium        • Procainamide
*Consider buffers.*

Resume attempts to defibrillate.

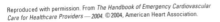

Stat!

## Asystole algorithm

---

**Primary ABCD survey**
*Focus: Basic CPR and defibrillation*

- Check responsiveness.
- Activate emergency response system.
- Call for defibrillator.
- **A**irway: Open the airway.
- **B**reathing: Provide positive-pressure ventilations.

- **C**irculation: Give chest compressions.
- **C**irculation: Confirm true asystole.
- **D**efibrillation: Assess for VF or pulseless VT; defibrillate, if indicated.
- Rapid scene survey: Any evidence personnel shouldn't attempt resuscitation?

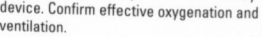

**Secondary ABCD survey**
*Focus: Advanced assessments and treatments*

- **A**irway: Place airway device and secure.
- **B**reathing: Confirm placement of airway device. Confirm effective oxygenation and ventilation.

- **C**irculation: Confirm true asystole. Establish I.V. access. Monitor rhythm. Give appropriate drugs.
- **D**ifferential diagnosis.

*Transcutaneous pacing*
If considered, perform immediately.

Epinephrine I.V. push

Atropine I.V. push

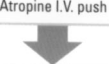

*Asystole persists*
Withhold or cease resuscitation efforts?
- Consider quality of resuscitation?
- Atypical clinical features present?
- Support for cease-efforts protocols in place?

## Selected references

*AHFS Drug Information 2005.* Bethesda, Md.: American Society of Health-System Pharmacists, Inc., 2005.

*Drug Facts and Comparisons,* 59th ed. Philadelphia: Lippincott Williams & Wilkins, 2005.

Evans-Smith, P. *Lippincott's Atlas of Medication Administration,* 2nd ed. Philadelphia: Lippincott Williams & Wilkins, 2005.

*ISMP Medication Safety Alert!* Huntingdon Valley, Pa.: Institute for Safe Medication Practice, 2004.

Karch, A. *Focus on Nursing Pharmacology,* 3rd ed. Philadelphia: Lippincott Williams & Wilkins, 2005.

*Medication Administration Made Incredibly Easy.* Philadelphia: Lippincott Williams & Wilkins, 2003.

*Nursing Pharmacology Made Incredibly Easy.* Philadelphia: Lippincott Williams & Wilkins, 2005.

*Nursing2006 Drug Handbook.* Philadelphia: Lippincott Williams & Wilkins, 2006.

"Patient Safety Guidelines," in *Comprehensive Accreditation Manual for Hospitals: The Official Handbook.* Oakbrook Terrace, Ill.: Joint Commission on Accreditation of Healthcare Organizations, 2005.

*Physicians' Desk Reference,* 58th ed. Oradell, N.J.: Medical Economics Company, 2004.

Roach, S. *Pharmacology for Health Professionals.* Philadelphia: Lippincott Williams & Wilkins, 2005.

## F

## G

## XY

## Z

## W